Making Markets for Vaccines
Ideas to action

The report of the
Center for Global Development
Advance Market Commitment Working Group

**Ruth Levine, Michael Kremer,
Alice Albright, Co-Chairs**

ISBN: 1-9332-8602-4

Library of Congress Cataloging-in-Publication Data
A catalog record has been requested

Editing, design and production by Bruce Ross-Larson, Christopher Trott, Timothy Walker and Elaine Wilson of Communications Development Incorporated, Washington, D.C., and Grundy & Northedge, London.

Lead report authors
Owen Barder
Michael Kremer
Ruth Levine

Working Group chairs
Alice Albright, The Vaccine Fund
Michael Kremer, Harvard University and Brookings Institution
Ruth Levine, Center for Global Development

Working Group members
Abhijit Banerjee, Massachusetts Institute of Technology
Amie Batson, World Bank
Ernst Berndt, Sloan School of Management, Massachusetts Institute of Technology
Lael Brainard, The Brookings Institution
David Cutler, Harvard University
David Gold, Global Health Strategies
Peter Hutt, Covington & Burling
Randall Kroszner, University of Chicago
Tom McGuire, Harvard University Medical School
Tomas Philipson, University of Chicago
Leighton Read, Alloy Ventures
Tom Scholar, U.K. Executive Director of International Monetary Fund & World Bank
Raj Shah, Bill & Melinda Gates Foundation
David Stephens, Emory University
Wendy Taylor, BIO Ventures for Global Health
Adrian Towse, Office of Health Economics
Sean Tunis, U.S. Department of Health and Human Services
Sharon White, U.K. Department for International Development
Victor Zonana, Global Health Strategies

Legal Advisors: John Hurvitz, with assistance from Stuart Irvin and Kevin Fisher, Covington & Burling

Staff: Gargee Ghosh (to July 2004)

Table of contents

Boxes

Figures

Tables

Preface

"He who receives an idea from me, receives instruction himself without lessening mine; as he who lights his taper at mine, receives light without darkening me. That ideas should freely spread from one to another over the globe, for the moral and mutual instruction of man, and improvement of his condition, seems to have been peculiarly and benevolently designed by nature..."

—Thomas Jefferson, August 13, 1813

In the time it takes you to read this preface, 100 people will die of diseases that can already be prevented with vaccines, and 150 more will die of malaria, HIV or tuberculosis.

If American or European children were dying at a rate of an average-sized high school every hour, it would lead the news every day. We would be devoting serious resources to finding a cure urgently.

But the people who die are too poor to command that sort of attention. Just 10% of the world's research and development on health is targeted on diseases affecting 90% of the world's people. Of more than a thousand new medicines developed over the last 25 years, just 1% were specifically for diseases of tropical countries.

There is not enough research and development because technological progress is a global public good. In the case of tropical diseases, no single individual enterprise has an incentive to pay for the full costs of developing new medicines. As a result, we invest far too little as a global community.

Nation-states have developed institutions, however imperfect, to invest in public goods, and these mutual commitments form part of the fabric of society. Nations provide security and financial stability, enforce contracts, protect the environment, limit inequality and poverty and invest in knowledge that enriches all their citizens. No doubt most countries could do these things better, but even so the provision of these common goods underpins the domestic social contract.

At the global level, by contrast, we lack institutions capable of providing and protecting global public goods. We have only sketchy arrangements to improve international security and maintain financial stability and little or nothing to preserve the environment, to provide a safety net against poverty or to invest in technological progress that would benefit all humanity. We lack adequate mechanisms to deliver a global social contract, in which those who can afford it make a fair contribution to the global society in which they live.

It is the poor who suffer most from the lack of public goods. While the rich can to some extent insulate themselves through private affluence, the poor shoulder the burden of public penury. Of course, the rich cannot shield themselves completely: in the long run, global public penury leads to an endless battle against illegal immigration, spread of infectious disease, proliferation of weapons, organized crime and drugs and spillovers of conflict.

Our failure to invest in the global commons flows not from our indifference but from our impotence, because we do not have incentives or mechanisms to coordinate our efforts to invest.

We at the Center for Global Development have sought ways to attack this problem—to strengthen the mechanisms, the incentives and the institutions that could underpin a more comprehensive global social contract.

Nowhere are the potential benefits greater than in the production and distribution of new vaccines to prevent the diseases that needlessly take lives and destroy livelihoods in developing countries.

In 2003 we established a Working Group, including economists, public health professionals, lawyers, experts in public policy and pharmaceutical and biotech experts, with the mandate to develop a practical approach to the vaccine challenge: to go from ideas to action. The result is this report.

My colleagues propose an elegant solution to enable the high-income countries to work together to accelerate the development of vaccines for diseases of low-income countries—to guarantee to pay for such vaccines if and when they are developed. The solution is simple and practical. It unleashes the same combination of market incentives and public investment that creates medicines for diseases that afflict us: arrangements that have been spectacularly effective in improving the health of the rich nations in the last century. It creates incentives for more private investment in these diseases. And it will ensure that, once a vaccine is developed, the funds will be there to get the vaccine to the people who need it.

Adequate investment in global public goods should be a cornerstone of foreign assistance. By definition, we all benefit from global public goods, and we share a responsibility to see that they are properly funded and available to everyone. These are investments with high returns and low risks of corruption and appropriation. Furthermore, this proposal ties funding directly to results: if the commitment does not succeed, there is no cost to the sponsors.

Every so often, an idea comes along that makes you ask: *now why didn't I think of that?* This is such an idea.

Nancy Birdsall
President
Center for Global Development
April 2005

Acknowledgments

This work would have been impossible without the contributions of many dedicated individuals. The Working Group chairs are deeply grateful to the members of the Advance Market Commitment Working Group, who spent two years exploring in detail whether and how an advanced market commitment could lead to faster development of desperately needed health products for the developing world. The Working Group brought diverse expertise and a unified commitment: to develop a practical proposal, one that would have the potential to transform the risk-benefit calculus for industry, donors and developing countries. Working Group members are profiled in appendix C.

We would like to thank the many individuals who offered comments on this and earlier drafts of the report and the term sheets, coming from the pharmaceutical and biotech industry and academic, global public health, policy and investor communities. Those comments helped us think (and rethink) both the rationale and the elements of such a commitment; they challenged and enriched our understanding of the ways in which different types of funding are needed to support the steps on the way to effective—and effectively delivered—vaccines; and they contributed to a more complete conception of the benefits and risks of purchase and price guarantees. (A list of individuals consulted appears in appendix D.)

We are particularly grateful for the opportunity provided by Charles Clift to engage in an e-consultation under the auspices of the Commission on Intellectual Property Rights, Innovation and Public Health in November and December 2004. We appreciate the comments of participants at the October 2004 meeting of the International Federation of Pharmaceutical Manufacturers Association; several Global Alliance for Vaccines and Immunization Financing Task Force meetings; the September 2003 malaria meeting in Mozambique; the 6th International Rotovirus Symposium in Mexico City in July 2004; and the March 2005 Malaria Vaccine Technology Roadmap meeting in Provence, France. None of those who commented are responsible in any way for the ultimate content of this report.

We appreciate the time and encouragement of Melinda Moree and the staff of the Malaria Vaccine Initiative and Seth Berkley and the staff of the International AIDS Vaccine Initiative. Generous with their knowledge and candid with their critiques, these individuals have strengthened this work greatly, but bear no responsibility for its ultimate content.

Several individuals made particularly important contributions to background analyses. We are indebted to Eyal Dvir, Rachel Glennerster, Jean Nahrae Lee, Julie Milstien, Violaine Mitchell, Rachel Podolsky, J. Niels Rosenquist, Georg Weizsacker and Heidi Williams. Their contributions are woven throughout this report.

Gargee Ghosh, who served as project manager from May 2003 through July 2004, deserves much of the credit for the group's progress through to the October 2004 consultation draft of this report, which was widely circulated. We are grateful for her strong analysis, skillful management and helpful impatience. Nancy Birdsall and other colleagues at the Center for Global Development have provided useful comments and advice throughout.

We thank the Bill & Melinda Gates Foundation for financial support for this work, and Raj Shah, Hannah Kettler, Gina Rabinovich, Rick Klausner and others at the Foundation for their active engagement throughout the project.

Finally, we are profoundly indebted to John Hurvitz, a partner of Covington & Burling, where he is co-chair of the firm's Life Sciences Industry Group and chair of the firm's Technology Transitions Group. Together with his colleagues Stuart Irvin and Kevin Fisher, John provided support of incomparable value throughout this project. He worked tirelessly under a pro bono arrangement to develop creative and practical solutions to thorny contractual problems, and effectively translated among the languages (and cultures) of law, business and public health. This generous contribution, provided out of a commitment to make the world a better place, is at the very heart of our report.

Policy highlights

Making a commitment in advance to buy vaccines if and when they are developed would create incentives for industry to increase investment in research and development (R&D). New commercial investment would complement funding of R&D by public and charitable bodies, accelerating the development of vital new vaccines for the developing world.

This report takes the proposal from theory to practice by showing how a commitment can be consistent with ordinary legal and budgetary principles. A draft contract term sheet is included, highlighting the key elements of a credible guarantee.

This generation can leave an historic legacy. By creating arrangements that spur the same scientific effort to diseases of the poor as we put into diseases of the rich, we can make a lasting contribution to the defeat of poverty.

Let our legacy be the conquest of disease:

- Barely 10% of global R&D is devoted to diseases that affect 90% of the world's population. AIDS, tuberculosis and malaria kill about 5 million people each year, yet we have no effective vaccine for these diseases—nor for others that primarily affect the poorest of the world's citizens.
- An advance market commitment would complement public and philanthropic funding of R&D and accelerate the development and availability of vaccines for diseases occurring mainly in the developing world. It would stimulate the allocation of commercial research funds to neglected diseases, and so harness the energy, experience and expertise of the private sector. Without a commitment, there will continue to be insufficient funding to bring more than a few, if any, candidate vaccines to market.
- Structured correctly, an advance market commitment could help to ensure both a reliable future supply of new vaccine products and affordable prices over the long term. There are good examples—discussed in chapter 2—of where similar incentives

have been effective; and the example of medicines for affluent countries demonstrates that, if the market is sufficiently valuable, there will be commercial investment in R&D.
- This commitment can be implemented in practice. It is based on sound and familiar legal principles that permit the rules—price, eligibility criteria and dispute resolution procedures—to be transparent and binding from the outset. The report includes draft contract term sheets that show how it can be done.
- For products at relatively early stages in their development, a commitment of $3 billion for each priority disease—an amount that would be comparable with sales of medicines in rich countries—would be a very good deal for the sponsors: a bargain compared with other development interventions, each life-year saved would cost less than $15.
- With appropriate contractual arrangements, the commitment would be applicable both to products at a late stage of development (such as vaccines against rotavirus and pneumococcus) and to products at an early stage (vaccines to prevent the transmission or mitigate the impact of malaria, HIV and tuberculosis).
- Both public and private philanthropic funders could make binding commitments within existing budgetary processes consistent with current regulatory and procurement systems for vaccines that would reach the poorest countries of the developing world.
- The commitment itself has no cost unless and until a vaccine is developed. It can be made without reducing the resources available to support health education and prevention, to buy existing vaccines and drugs, to strengthen health systems in developing countries or to fund R&D and public-private partnerships. Funding for these high priority activities can, and should, be increased in the short term. These are important complements to increased commercial investment in R&D.
- Progress will be accelerated if we do more to buy existing vaccines. It is essential to boost and strengthen vaccination

delivery systems in developing countries, to improve demand forecasts and to extend long-term procurement for existing vaccines. These measures would save lives today—and complement an advance market commitment by making the market for vaccines larger and more certain.

- Scientific breakthroughs are by no means the answer to all the problems of poor countries. But they can play, and have played in the past, a major role in improving the health of those who have the least. Building on the achievements of the past, this generation of scientists could find ways to prevent malaria and tuberculosis, stop the spread of HIV/AIDS and dramatically reduce the toll on children of diarrhoeal and respiratory disease. But such accomplishments are unlikely to happen without incentives that take such work out of the exclusive realm of altruism and charity, and place it squarely in the domain of functioning, sustainable markets, creating incentives for the private sector to bring the full weight of its experience and assets to bear.

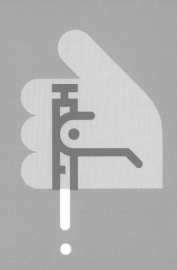

Summary
A legacy
of our
generation

This generation has a unique opportunity to leave a legacy of which we can be proud. Current and near-future scientific knowledge can be used to conquer diseases that kill millions of people each year and disable millions more. In the development of vaccines, in particular, scientific breakthroughs have the potential to transform the health of the developing world much as they have been instrumental in almost eliminating the burden of life-threatening infectious disease among children in affluent nations. The most significant challenges are ahead: we have not yet developed effective vaccines against diseases of the poor, such as malaria, HIV and tuberculosis.

Governments and private foundations have made enormous strides in recent years toward establishing arrangements that will facilitate investment in R&D needed to develop new vaccines for these diseases. Now the resources and talent of the private sector are needed to translate those investments, and the scientific breakthroughs they are producing, into new vaccines, which once developed would be manufactured in adequate quantity. Unfortunately, the absence of an adequate market for those vaccines makes it impossible for the private sector to make investments in these diseases on a commercially viable basis.

We could make it worthwhile for the pharmaceutical industry to invest much more in R&D on vaccines for diseases occurring mainly in developing countries—and in the mass production of those vaccines when they have been developed. This can be done simply and cheaply by ensuring that there is a market for the vaccines if and when they become available.

Why vaccines: The unrealized potential of immunization

Immunization has had a profound impact on global health, in rich countries as well as poor. Immunization is cheap, reliable and effective, and is reaching the majority of children in low-income countries. But we have not capitalized on the full potential that immunization offers. Many more lives in the developing world could be saved and improved with increased access to existing and new vaccines.

First, we need to improve the availability of existing vaccines. That 3 million people die every year of diseases that can be prevented with existing vaccines is evidence of a profound failure in the current system. This failure can be remedied with more predictable financial resources, stronger political commitment to

public health, greater investment in both immunization-specific and broader elements of health systems and better management at all levels, global to local.

Second, we need to accelerate the development of new vaccines targeted to and appropriate for the epidemiological conditions and health systems of developing countries. Part of the solution lies in establishing secure financing for the medium term so that countries are willing to introduce vaccines that cost more than the "pennies per dose" that ministries of health (and donors) have come to expect. Another part of the solution is to ensure sufficient funding and the right incentives for innovation to develop new health technologies, both in the short and long term. Given the range of what is needed—investment in basic science, conduct of clinical trials, development of new manufacturing capabilities for cutting-edge products and scaling up of manufacturing over the long term—these incentives should be designed to attract investment by private firms of many types: biotechnology firms, multinational pharmaceutical companies and emerging suppliers, including in developing countries such as India.

Intensive and growing efforts are being directed along many but not all of the necessary fronts:

- The Global Alliance on Vaccines and Immunization's (GAVI) recent investments in vaccines and strengthening health care systems, along with the long-standing efforts of national governments and international donors.
- The International Finance Facility for Immunization initiative (IFFIm) and other efforts seeking to establish an adequate and predictable funding base.
- GAVI's Accelerated Development and Introduction Plans (ADIPs) to generate information for good decisionmaking about introducing new products.
- Increased funding for research on neglected diseases, for example through product development public-private partnerships as well as traditional publicly funded research.

These efforts are beginning to show results with improvements in immunization coverage and introduction of newer vaccines, as well as the accumulation of scientific knowledge and the development of promising new vaccine candidates. But one dimension of the problem has gone largely unaddressed by policymakers: the lack of market-based incentives for pharmaceutical companies to complement these existing efforts with the R&D necessary to move promising vaccine candidates from the lab through to scaled-up manufacturing.

New medicines are a shared endeavor

Developing a new vaccine or drug is expensive because of formidable scientific challenges and stringent regulatory requirements.[1] Candidate medicines must be tested, first in small and then in large trials. Regulatory approval must be obtained. Investment is needed in manufacturing and distribution capacity, meeting a high standard for safety and quality. Estimates of the total cost of developing a new medicine vary from hundreds of millions of dollars to well over $1 billion.

For most medicines available today, this investment has been financed by a mixture of public funding by government, philanthropic and charitable giving and private investment. Firms make those investments in R&D with the expectation of being able to sell the finished product for a profit and so recover their investment.

For health conditions that affect affluent countries, basic scientific development is the result of a mixture of publicly funded research in tandem with a more limited amount of commercial investment in basic science. The later stages of product development, including clinical trials, approval and manufacturing—stages that make up more than two-thirds of the total costs of developing new medicines—are funded primarily by commercial pharmaceutical companies. While nearly all medicines depend to some extent on publicly funded science, the private sector is the single largest funder of medical R&D, and typically takes on the challenge of converting scientific advances into usable products. Those costs are then passed on to the consumers and governments, directly or through insurance.

It is difficult to overstate the importance of commercial investment in medicine. Market incentives are particularly effective in ensuring that R&D is targeted at strategies that will bring the best possible products to market as quickly as possible.

A piece of the puzzle is missing

Commercial biotech and pharmaceutical companies have to target their R&D on products that will produce a commercial return; this usually means medicines for the high-value markets of high-income countries. As things stand today, the markets for vaccines and drugs for diseases occurring mainly in developing countries are not valuable enough to offer sufficient returns to provide commercial justification for the necessary expensive research and product development.

So for health conditions that primarily affect poor countries, there is little or no commercial investment to complement publicly financed R&D. An estimated 10% of the world's R&D investment is in solutions for diseases that affect 90% of the world's people.[2] Even where public investment results in promising scientific leads, limited resources mean that many of those leads languish in the laboratory, with insufficient resources and few champions to bring more than a few of them through to the next, more expensive stages of product development and clinical trials.

Commercial investment would accelerate new medicines

The prospects for R&D for products that would prevent or treat diseases concentrated in developing countries has been significantly improved in recent years by the establishment of partnerships[3] that, largely through funding from philanthropic foundations such as the Rockefeller Foundation and the Bill & Melinda Gates Foundation, have greatly increased the resources available to accelerate the development of medicines for developing countries.

While these efforts have vastly enhanced the prospects for finding vaccines for these diseases, resources are still too small to fund the development of more than a small number of candidate medicines. Moreover, incentives for the full engagement of the private sector, which will be essential for efficient scale-up and manufacture, are not in place. The result is slow progress through clinical trials and the commercial development of new vaccines, and potentially a premature narrowing of the field of candidates. Were it available, commercial funding would increase the number of products under development and accelerate clinical trials, and so raise the chances of success for second-generation products and a greater diversity of new vaccines. This is particularly important in the case of malaria and AIDS, where the first-to-market vaccine may be only partially efficacious, and there will be a strong need to push the science further.

We can create incentives for commercial investment

Incentives for commercial investment in R&D and manufacturing can be created through an advance market commitment, in which donors make a legally binding pledge to pay for a new vaccine, if and when one is developed (box 1).[4] Such a commitment would create a larger and more certain market. It would imitate the market conditions that stimulate research for diseases common in developed countries. It would create incentives for more firms to identify and pursue promising avenues of research and to compete to bring them to market as quickly as possible. It would attract firms to develop new products for these diseases.

Such a commitment would enable donors to increase the incentives for commercial investment without reducing the resources available for immediate investment in R&D through public-private partnerships and other existing arrangements.

Create a market not a prize

The Center for Global Development Advance Market Commitment Working Group has designed an advance market

---

Box 1
The main features of the proposed commitment

- An agreed technical specification—in terms of outputs—required of a new vaccine.
- A price guarantee, consisting of small payments from eligible countries and a co-payment by sponsors, would apply to a maximum number of treatments. (For example, the price might be guaranteed at $15 per treatment, with the eligible low-income country paying $1 and sponsors topping up the payment with an additional $14 for the first 200 million treatments.)
- An overall market size of about $3 billion—enough to make it worthwhile for firms to accelerate investment in research and development for new vaccines, but well below the social value of the vaccine.
- An independent adjudication committee to oversee the arrangements and commitments enforceable under the law.
- In return for taking up the guaranteed price on the first treatments sold, the producer would be obliged to commit to produce and sell further treatments in eligible countries at a fixed, low sustainable price.
- Total sales of each qualifying product would depend on demand from developing countries. This in turn would depend on the effectiveness of the vaccine and the available alternatives.

---

commitment that would be practical and effective. It would create a market, not a prize, and so avoid some of the pitfalls of a "winner-take-all" mechanism.

The main elements of our findings are that:

- A legally binding commitment can be made within the conventional framework of existing contract law (we include draft contract term sheets to illustrate the arrangement).
- Government donors can make this commitment within existing budget processes; it would have no impact on public spending unless and until a vaccine is developed.
- Government and philanthropic investments in research and the creation of an advance market commitment are mutually reinforcing, collectively accelerating progress.
- A market of approximately $3 billion for each priority disease for which substantial R&D is needed would create revenues comparable in value with revenues that firms obtain for pharmaceutical products in affluent countries.
- For diseases that impose the largest health burden on developing countries, the cost of vaccines under such a commitment would be outstanding value for money for donors, more cost-effective than almost any existing development assistance. Purchases under an advance market commitment for a malaria vaccine are roughly estimated to cost less than $15 life-year saved.
- Consistent with current thinking in development assistance and aid effectiveness, payments are linked to results. If a commitment is put in place and no vaccine is developed, there will be no financial cost. If such a commitment succeeds, millions of lives will be saved at very low cost.
- This would create a set of incentives comparable to those that exist for diseases of high-income countries. Firms would be likely to respond to a commitment by increasing investment in R&D and scaling up production capacity, thereby accelerating the development of new vaccines, increasing competition and fostering long-term affordability.

Benefits to developing countries, donors and industry

Carefully designed advance market commitments can offer substantial benefits to donors, industry and—most importantly—developing countries. For donors, this is a low-risk, transparent, cost-effective investment that guarantees widespread access to vaccines if and when they are developed. In this results-oriented approach, there is a financial cost to sponsors only if a vaccine is developed. In addition, the structure of these commitments guarantees that this would be a financially sustainable donor investment. For industry, an advance market commitment creates a risk-reward structure with which firms are already familiar: they will be rewarded if they bring to market a product for which there is real demand. Unlike many alternative proposals, access issues are addressed without weakening incentives or dismantling the system of intellectual property rights. Most important, for developing countries an advance market commitment is likely to significantly accelerate the development and distribution of essential vaccines, of great value to sustainably improving the health of people in poor countries. The commitment ensures that, if a new vaccine is developed, it will be rapidly available in developing countries at an affordable price.

Next steps

We recommend that donors, industry and the public health community work together to develop an advance market commitment for critical diseases occurring mainly in developing countries, including (but not necessarily limited to) HIV, tuberculosis and malaria. In doing this, we recommend further and more targeted analytic work by governments, industry and public health experts on several key topics.

Priorities for further work include:

- Strengthening financing for the purchase of existing vaccines, and strengthening health systems in developing countries to increase vaccine coverage.
- Developing long-term advance market commitments with producers of vaccines that will be available in the near future, using the commitment to negotiate on price, timing

of supply and characteristics of the vaccines and their presentation.

For vaccines that are at an early stage:

- Considering the specific issues with respect to individual diseases (such as the likely demand from high-income and middle-income markets).
- Validating our estimates of the market size needed to induce private sector investment in R&D, using alternative datasets for market revenues.
- Working closely with industry and the public health community to develop the contractual framework, including addressing the various design choices highlighted here.
- Developing technical specifications for each product, in collaboration with developing country health specialists and the scientific community.
- Considering what adaptations, if any, should be made to mechanisms for funding R&D in the context of an advance market commitment.
- Considering how this approach might be extended to other diseases that affect the developing world, such as schistosomiasis or leishmaniasis, and for drugs and medical diagnostics.

This report lays out the rationale for this approach. More important, it sets out a blueprint for implementation.

We have been heartened and impressed by the speed of policymakers in responding to the Consultation Draft of our report. Policy processes are now in place to establish a commitment for such diseases as malaria and HIV. We fully acknowledge that there is more work to be done, and that the Working Group's ideas will likely require modification as they are put into practice. We hope that this report will encourage the continuing discussion between donors, industry and the public health community in agreeing on the details of advance market commitments.

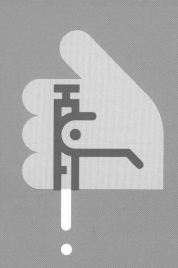

1
We need to invest more in vaccines

Chapter at a glance

- Vaccines represent the best hope for large, rapid and affordable improvements in health in the developing world.
- Vaccines developed for affluent countries have already contributed greatly to improving the health of people in poor countries. A remarkable 75% of children receive a basic set of childhood immunizations. But because of shortcomings in financing and delivery, including delays in introduction of life-saving vaccines, more than 3 million people die each year of vaccine-preventable diseases.
- Increasingly, the main diseases in poor countries are not a high priority in affluent countries. As a result, developing countries can no longer depend on rich markets to meet the costs of the development of new vaccines that would benefit poor countries.
- The total market size for vaccines in developing countries is tiny— about $500 million a year. This is insufficient to provide an incentive for pharmaceutical companies to invest in developing new vaccines for these diseases.
- In addition to being small, the vaccine market is characterized by collective procurement. Success in stretching health budgets by keeping prices as low as possible has important short-term benefits. But the aim of minimizing short-term costs to ensure access must be balanced with the goal of providing returns sufficient to stimulate development of new products.
- Largely as a result of the low value and high risks of the developing country market, less than 10% of global spending on health research and development is devoted to the major health problems of 90% of the population.
- Without a valuable market to stimulate the development of new vaccines for diseases that occur mainly in developing countries, alternative arrangements are needed to ensure that vaccines are developed, produced on a large scale and made available affordably and reliably to developing countries.

1

We need to invest more in vaccines

Vaccines are important for global health

The importance of the development of new vaccines for the most significant health problems in the developing world can hardly be overstated. Well known as being among the most cost-effective health interventions, immunization can be cost-saving, by preventing diseases that would otherwise require expensive treatment. In general, vaccines are well suited to the needs of developing countries. They are a cheap way to save lives, requiring no costly screening, diagnosis or follow-up.

Extraordinary scientific progress, coupled with effective delivery strategies, has transformed health conditions in the past 50 years, in both rich and poor countries. In the industrial world, for example, basic childhood immunization has almost eliminated many diseases that once crippled, severely sickened or killed thousands of young children each year (figure 1.1).[1]

Those same vaccines—originally developed for the United States and Europe—have been used in the developing world, typically sold at low prices after manufacturing capacity had expanded. These low prices are possible because the developers of the vaccines have been able to earn a return on their investment from sales in affluent countries. As patent protection has come to an end, and the markets have become contestable, production volumes have increased and the prices charged to developing countries have fallen close to the marginal cost of production, a few cents. For example, the combined diphtheria, tetanus and pertussis (DTP) vaccine costs about $0.09 a dose, and the measles vaccine costs about $0.14 a dose.

Even with lower levels of coverage than in developed countries, these products have had an enormous health impact in the developing world. More than three-quarters of the world's children receive the basic childhood immunizations.

Vaccines have transformed global health. Smallpox used to kill 5 million people a year; thanks to the world's first vaccine, it was eradicated in 1979 (box 1.1). Fifty years ago, polio was the leading cause of paralysis, crippling thousands of children and adults. The eradication of polio through vaccination is tantalizingly close, though it will require continuing focus and commitment from policymakers. Two-thirds of developing countries have eliminated neonatal tetanus. In one year alone (from June 2001) mass measles campaigns in eight African countries vaccinated more than 20 million children and prevented more than 140,000 deaths; measles vaccinations are now preventing 250,000 deaths

Figure 1.1
Basic childhood immunizations reduce reported cases of disease in developed and developing countries—selected examples

Reported cases of measles, 1980–2000

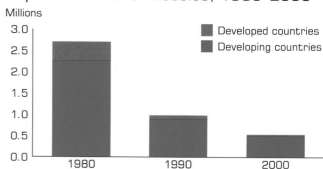

Reported cases of pertussis, 1980–2000

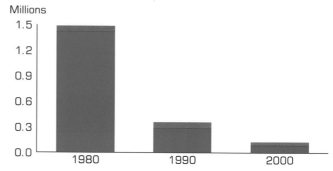

Reported cases of diphtheria, 1980–2000

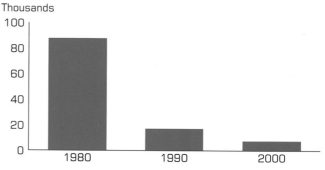

Source: WHO Immunization Profiles for Developed and Developing country groups.

a year.[2] As a result of both routine immunization programs and campaigns, millions of lives are saved every year; and millions more are protected from disease and disability.

Millions die of vaccine-preventable diseases

In many ways, it is extraordinary how effectively vaccines reach children all over the world. More than three-quarters of the world's children are vaccinated, and vaccines reach children in

Box 1.1
The eradication of smallpox

An estimated 300 million people died from smallpox in the 20th century. As a result of a global effort, financed in part by foreign aid, the disease has been eradicated.

In the middle of the 20th century there were approximately 10–15 million cases of smallpox in more than 50 countries, and 1.5–2 million people died of the disease each year. Smallpox killed about a third of the people it infected.

In 1965 international efforts to eradicate smallpox were revitalized by a new Smallpox Eradication Unit at the World Health Organization and a pledge for more technical and financial support from the campaign's largest donor, the United States. Endemic countries were supplied with vaccines and kits for collecting and sending specimens, and vaccination was made easier by the provision of bifurcated needles. An intensified effort was led in the five remaining countries in 1973, with the surveillance and containment of outbreaks. By 1977 the last endemic case of smallpox was recorded in Somalia. In May 1980, after two years of surveillance and searching, the World Health Assembly declared that smallpox was the first disease in history to have been eradicated.

The cost of the smallpox campaign between 1967 and 1979 was $23 million a year. International donors provided $98 million, while $200 million came from the affected countries.

Source: Levine and others (2004).

remote areas, overcoming formidable obstacles of geography, conflict and poverty.

Even so, about 3 million people a year die of diseases that can be prevented with existing vaccines, such as measles, hepatitis B and tetanus. People die of vaccine-preventable diseases partly because approximately 25% of children, almost all of them in developing countries, do not receive a full set of immunizations (figure 1.2). And those who are immunized do not always get newer vaccines against some high-risk diseases because, though suitable vaccines exist, cost and other barriers have delayed their widespread introduction.

Low-income countries have benefited from R&D investments made in response to the market in high- and middle-income countries; but vaccines developed for high-income markets have been introduced in developing countries only after a considerable delay—typically 10–15 years or more (figure 1.3). For example, during the 1990s the use of a vaccine for Hib[3] (a strain that causes some forms of pneumonia and meningitis) almost eliminated Hib-related diseases in high-income countries. But the vaccine remains too expensive for use in most low-income countries.[4] As a result, an estimated 4.5 million unvaccinated children died from Hib-related diseases—mainly pneumonia—over the last decade (see figure 1.2).[5] (Note that hepatitis B vaccination does

Figure 1.2
A million and a half children died from vaccine-preventable diseases in 2002

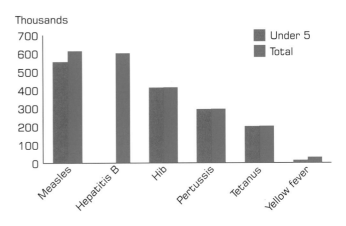

Source: WHO (2004c).

not prevent child deaths, but it prevents adult deaths if it is given to children early enough.)

More investment needed in vaccines for diseases concentrated in developing countries

Over and above the experience of delayed introduction of new products, desperately needed new vaccines simply may not be developed at all. Today, the health needs of children in the poorest countries are now quite different than those of children in Europe, Japan and the United States.

Fifteen years ago, a child born almost anywhere in the world received more or less the same basic vaccines—DTwP (diphtheria, tetanus and whole-cell pertussis [whooping cough]), OPV (oral polio vaccine) and BCG (tuberculosis).[6] Over time, however, as

major childhood killers like measles were conquered in wealthy countries, new vaccines that are quite specific to rich-world conditions were developed. In some cases, vaccines were enhanced to decrease the (already very low) risks of adverse reactions. In general, these vaccines are costlier to produce. As a result of these changes, a child born in the rich world today receives different vaccines than a child in the developing world (figure 1.4).[7]

The priority diseases for poor countries are not the main priorities for rich countries. AIDS is a leading cause of death in the low-income countries, but it is not even one of the top 10 killers in high-income countries. Diarrhoeal diseases, malaria and other childhood diseases also appear on the developing world's top 10 causes of death, but are nowhere on the equivalent list for rich countries. Communicable diseases are the cause of 56% of the disease burden in low-income countries, and just 6% of the disease burden in high-income countries (table 1.1). The target product characteristics are also different: heat stability, safety and affordability continue to be major concerns for the developing world, while the developed world is driving toward very low risk vaccines even if this substantially adds to the cost.

As the pharmaceutical industry has responded to the health needs of the world's better-off, diseases that are concentrated in the poorest populations have largely been neglected (see table 1.1). The spectrum of available vaccines, even if used comprehensively, would not solve the major health problems facing the developing world.

Figure 1.3
Years from availability in developing countries for hepatitis B and Hib

Millions of doses

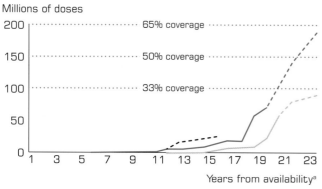

-----Hepatitis B, all developing countries

-----Hepatitis B, all developing countries, excluding China, India and Indonesia[b]

-----Hib, all developing countries[c]

a. Based on GAVI estimates for Vaccine Fund–eligible countries, plus countries that introduced the vaccine prior to GAVI. Last 5 years are estimates.

b. Excludes China, India or Indonesia because of the high uncertainty whether they will introduce the vaccine or because they may use it only if manufactured locally.

c. Coverage in all Vaccine Fund–eligible countries, including China, India and Indonesia (total of 95 million children).

Source: World Bank, Bill & Melinda Gates Foundation and GAVI (2002).

Figure 1.4
Vaccination gaps between children in rich and poor countries

Number of immunizations

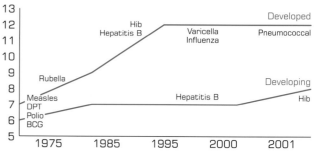

Source: Batson (2001).

AIDS, tuberculosis and malaria account for about 5 million deaths a year; there is no effective vaccine for any of these three diseases, and the science for each is at an early stage. Pneumococcus is estimated to kill 1.1 million people a year, and rotavirus 0.8 million. For pneumococcus, vaccines are being developed, but they will need to be adapted to protect against the serotypes that account for the burden of disease in developing countries (box 1.3). Even once vaccines have been licensed for use, previous experience suggests that it will be many years before they are widely available at prices affordable to most developing countries. The form of the disease

they protect against may not be the form that is most common in developing countries. Other diseases primarily affecting the developing world for which no vaccines are available include shigella, schistosomiasis, leishmaniasis, chagas disease and dengue.[8]

This means that the developing world's previous source of affordable vaccines—residual supply from the developed world, at tiered prices—is no longer a reliable model. When new products are developed with the rich world—not the poor—in mind, diseases concentrated in the developing world are left behind. Not only would vaccines suitable for the developing world reduce the burden of disease, but it is generally believed that these health improvements would have substantial positive impacts on economic growth and poverty reduction (WHO 2003c) (box 1.2).

Pharmaceutical development is a risky investment decision

R&D-based pharmaceutical companies and biotechnology firms are in a risky business. Their business model is to place smart

Table 1.1
Global burden of disease in 2002, disaggregated by cause

Cause	Percent of total world disease burden	Percent of total disease burden in high-income countries	Percent of total disease burden in low-income countries
Communicable, maternal and perinatal diseases	41.0	6.2	56.4
Infectious and parasitic diseases	23.9	2.5	34.1
HIV/AIDS	5.8	0.6	7.6
Tuberculosis	2.4	0.1	3.0
Malaria	3.0	0.0	4.9
Respiratory infections	6.1	1.2	8.4
Other	11.1	2.5	13.9
Noncommunicable conditions	46.7	84.7	32.6
Malignant neoplasms (cancers)	5.1	14.7	2.4
Cardiovascular diseases	9.9	15.3	7.3
Other	31.7	54.7	22.8
Injuries	12.2	9.1	11.0

Note: Figures are disability-adjusted life years (see chapter 5 for definition). Country classifications are from World Development Indicators (World Bank 2003), based on World Bank estimates of 2001 gross national income per capita. Data for upper- and lower-middle-income countries are not shown.

Source: WHO (2003c).

Box 1.2
Public health and economic growth

Public health matters because health measures offer the opportunity to save millions of lives and improve the quality of life for millions more. Many argue that improving health could also have a major impact on economic development, in part through a direct impact of increased life expectancy. Estimates are controversial, but one estimate by Jeffrey Sachs is that countries with intensive malaria grew 1.3% less per person a year; and that a 10% reduction in malaria was associated with 0.3% a year higher growth.[a] A study of the United States found that more than half the growth of real income in the first half of the 20th century was attributable to declining mortality.[b] In other words, reducing the burden of disease can make a direct contribution not only to achieving the health-related Millennium Development Goals, but more generally to the lives and prosperity of the developing world.

a. Gallup and Sachs (2000).

b. Nordhaus (2003).

bets on science in the face of imperfect market information. Firms get their competitive edge from doing this well. Vaccine development can take 7–20 years for basic research, clinical testing, regulatory approval, production and distribution—and at each of the stages, even the most promising candidates can fail to perform as hoped.

The investment costs are high. Estimates of the total cost vary, depending in part on what is measured. The range is from several hundred million dollars to more than $1.5 billion. One often-cited study finds a cost of $802 million for a new medicine, up to the point of regulatory approval.[9]

One reason that these estimated costs are so high is that these investments are uncertain: of all the candidate products that enter development, only a small proportion will be successful, and far fewer will become "blockbusters" that earn a significant return for the company. For vaccine companies to stay in business, each successful product has to recover not only the costs of its own design and development, but also the costs of the unsuccessful candidates.

The development of new products is, in effect, the outcome of a series of bets placed on emerging scientific pathways, based on a hard-nosed analysis of the competitive landscape and some reasonable estimates of the eventual market size and willingness to pay. The companies that do this best undertake their own research and work in partnership with biotech companies, research scientists, academics and others. The final product combines the

Box 1.3
Pneumococcus

The bacterium Streptococcus pneumoniae is the most common cause of severe pneumonia worldwide. It also causes meningitis, septicaemia and ear infections.

Although estimates of its death toll are made difficult by various factors, the pneumococcus bacterium (Streptococcus pneumoniae) is thought to kill 1.1 million people worldwide each year, most of them young children and infants.

In developing countries as many as 1 in 10 deaths in young children is attributed to this infection. Although vaccines for adults and children ages two and older have been available for years, they have not been suitable for the babies and toddlers who are most vulnerable to the disease because the current vaccines do not stimulate an appropriate immune response.

However, a new conjugate vaccine that is highly effective in infants has recently been approved for marketing by the Food and Drug Administration (FDA) in the United States, and several more vaccines are in late stages of development. But it is unclear whether these will be as effective in developing country settings as they are in developed countries.

Pneumococcal vaccines protect by stimulating antibodies against the specific polysaccharide (complex sugar) capsules that cover the bacteria. There are more than 80 specific pneumococcal capsular polysaccharides. The pneumococcal conjugate vaccine licensed by the FDA stimulates the production of protective antibodies against the seven serotypes that most frequently cause invasive disease in the United States. However, this "7-valent" vaccine does not stimulate antibodies against two serotypes, 1 and 5, which together are thought to be responsible for 12%–25% of invasive pneumococcal disease in many developing countries.

With such countries in mind, researchers and the vaccine industry have developed 9-valent and 11-valent pneumococcal conjugate vaccines that stimulate antibodies against serotypes 1 and 5. These vaccines are the subject of large-scale field trials in several countries in Africa, Asia and Latin America. Recommendations about the use of the new pneumococcal vaccines among infants in developing countries will depend on the results of these trials, the initial results of which have been spectacularly positive.

Source: GAVI (2005a).

scientific knowledge, innovation and intellectual property of a large number of partners.

Despite these uncertainties, the market for medicines in the developed world succeeds in generating important new products. Effective and innovative drugs and vaccines are invented, tested, licensed and produced. The functioning of the market for affluent countries depends on patents and regulatory protection, which grant the manufacturer a temporary period of market exclusivity. This means that manufacturers are able to charge consumers a price high enough not only to cover the cost of production but also the costs of research and development. Market considerations play an important part in each stage of the process as possible medicines move from investment in basic research, through to clinical trials, licensing, production and supply (figure 1.5).

By offering the opportunity to charge temporarily higher prices for the medicines, market exclusivity acts as a "pull" mechanism, providing pharmaceutical companies with sufficient incentive to make risky investments, some of which will eventually result in life-saving medicines of enormous social value.

The small market for vaccines for developing countries

The total market for vaccines for developing countries is about $500 million a year[10] (figure 1.6), though it is growing as a result of increased spending through GAVI, which has spent some $530 million since it was launched in 2000.[11]

Total spending on health in the least developed countries averages $17 a person a year, of which about $6 a person is from the country's government budget. For slightly better-off low-income countries, the average is about $36 a person a year.[12] (The equivalent figure for high-income countries is $2,263 a year.)

Figure 1.5
Vaccine development pipeline

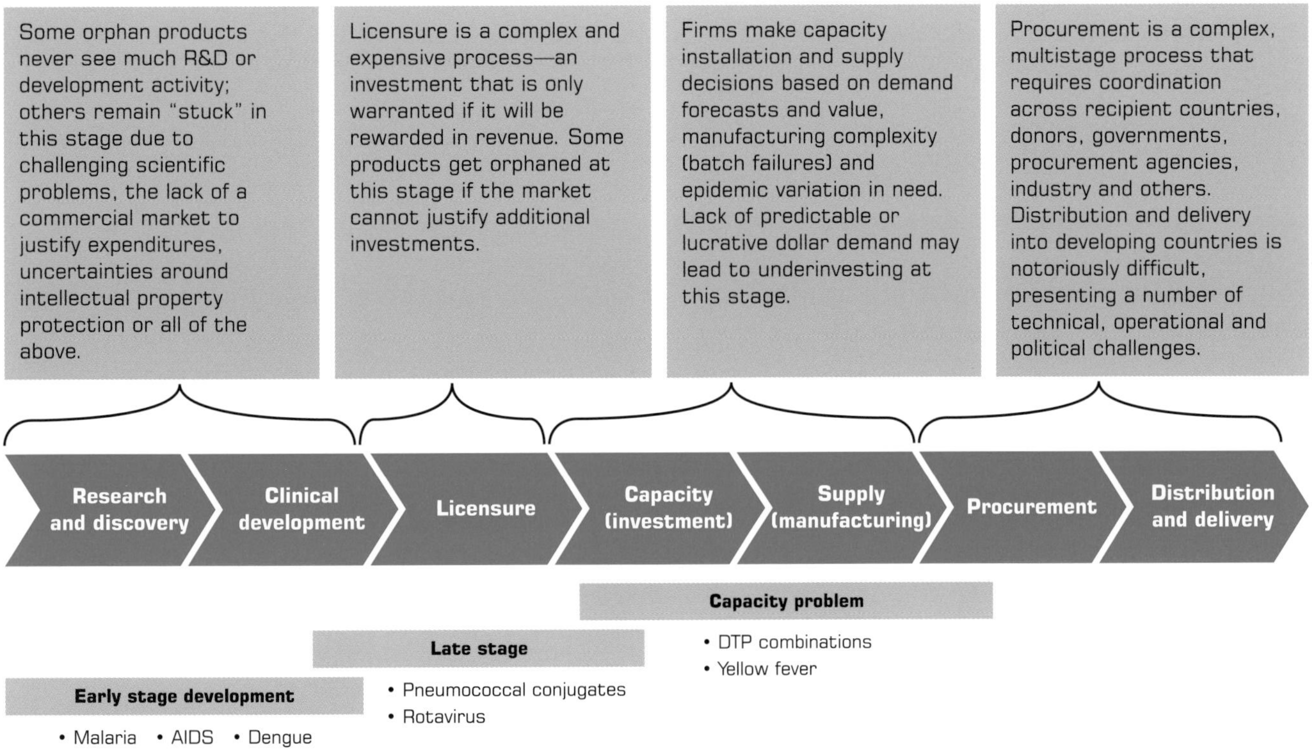

The differentials in health spending are reflected in the vaccine market. The global market for vaccines is about $6 billion a year—accounting for only 1.5% of global pharmaceutical sales.[13] Global sales of all vaccines combined are roughly equivalent to annual sales of a single blockbuster drug such as Lipitor or Prilosec.[14] Developing-country markets account for about half the total vaccine sales by volume, but provide only about 5%—or less—of total revenues from vaccine sales. So developing-country vaccines currently make up a negligible proportion—less than 0.1%—of the value of pharmaceutical sales.

Public procurement policies must balance long- and short-term interests

From a commercial perspective, the arrangements that developing countries and development agencies use to buy medicines may compound the problem of an anemic market size. Most vaccines are bought by public health authorities or on their behalf by the procurement divisions at agencies such as the United Nations Children's Fund (UNICEF). Once firms have sunk R&D resources on a vaccine, governments—in the interests of protecting scarce health budgets—have an incentive to use their role as dominant purchasers, regulators and arbiters of intellectual property rights to negotiate the lowest possible price. Given the very limited funds available for health, even with international donor support for immunization programs, achieving a low price

is an essential way for these authorities to buy valuable health products for as many people as possible.

But the short-term need to get vaccines to many people competes with the long-term need to ensure that firms can meet the costs of R&D and also provide returns to shareholders. This is particularly problematic when both developing-country governments and donor agencies have become accustomed to buying vaccines at "pennies per dose." Buying vaccines at very low prices means that firms receive little more than the cost of production, not enough to recover the costs of the original R&D. Knowing in advance that buyers will want to push prices down in this way, it is difficult for firms to plan to invest in these products at all.

Uncertainties in demand, in addition to the monopsony, increase the risks. International agencies' procurement arrangements typically do not bind the purchaser to buy the full number of doses for which tenders are issued. The quantity purchased may be much less than expected because of unforeseen calamities, volatility in the availability of donor or domestic funding, weak information systems and many other shortcomings in the ability to forecast demand. Given nonbinding contractual arrangements, the quantity risk lies entirely with the supplier.

The need to reduce the lag time

Pooled procurement and uncertain demand are not the only factors that create an unfavorable risk-reward profile. Increasingly, activists and public-policy makers are unwilling to accept long lag times between the availability of life-saving drugs in the rich countries and access to those products at prices affordable to developing countries. The pressure on donors and firms to make antiretroviral drugs available to those with HIV/AIDS has brought this issue into sharp relief, but it is also the topic of active debate in the immunization field.

Pharmaceutical firms know when they are planning future research that, once a medicine is available, governments will wish to negotiate the price down and the company will come under pressure from public opinion to make important medicines available as cheaply as possible. In extreme cases, the developer of an essential new medicine may face compulsory licensing. If the firm does not expect to be able to recover its development costs at the price it will able to charge, it will hesitate to invest in developing the medicine in the first place.[15] As one senior industry executive

Figure 1.6
Markets for vaccines are much smaller than those for pharmaceuticals

Annual revenue (billions of dollars)

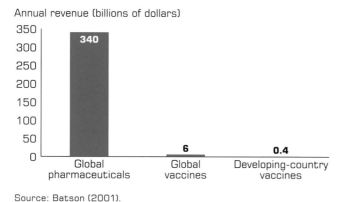

Source: Batson (2001).

said, "Our worst nightmare would be to discover a vaccine for AIDS. We would be forced to give it away."

With no valuable market, the prospects for the development of new vaccines to prevent or mitigate the severity of disease concentrated in low-income countries through innovation in the private sector are not promising. As we shall see in chapter 2, only 13 (1%) of the new chemical entities brought to market from 1975 to 1997 were specifically for diseases of developing countries; and of these, only 4 were the direct results of R&D activities of the pharmaceutical industry targeted at new human products.[16] While there is some modest commercial investment, we are some way away from providing incentives that would engage the full resources and energy of the pharmaceutical and biotech firms in finding these solutions, which are essential to improving human health.

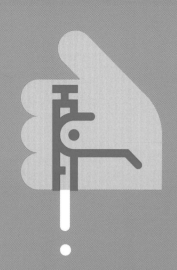

2

Promoting private investment in vaccine development

Chapter at a glance

- The development of a new medicine depends on the work of scientists based in academic, government and private research institutions, focusing on challenges that range from understanding a particular type of immune response to determining what type of packaging will maintain the viability of heat-sensitive products.
- Commercial investment is complemented in essential ways by public and philanthropic funding, which is especially important for the basic science and early-stage research on which pharmaceutical development depends. But the most expensive, later stages of vaccine development—such as clinical testing, regulatory approval, production and distribution—are mainly the result of private sector investment.
- For drugs and vaccines that are produced for populations in affluent countries, the single largest source of funding for R&D is commercial investment.[1]

- R&D on products that address health problems in developing countries receives neither the level nor the type of funding that health problems in developed countries receive. Of more than $100 billion spent on health R&D across the world, only about $6 billion is spent each year on diseases of developing countries, almost all of which is from public and philanthropic sources. There is little commercial investment because the market is not large enough to provide financial returns to cover the costs.
- A number of different approaches can be used to make investments in neglected diseases more attractive— and some have already been tried in a limited context and have demonstrated a positive effect.
- An advance market commitment would have important benefits:
  - First, it would mobilize additional resources, particularly for the clinical testing phases of development.

- Second, strong market incentives would mobilize the ingenuity, energy, intellectual assets and managerial capacity of the pharmaceutical sector—from biotechs to multinational firms.
  - Third, it would allow public sector and philanthropic funders to stand at arm's length from complex scientific choices and tradeoffs, allowing firms to make their own judgments about the scientific feasibility and risks of alternative strategies.
  - Fourth, it would pay only for results, providing sponsors with the assurance that large-scale funding would be provided if and only if an effective and safe product that is appropriate for the developing world is manufactured in large enough quantity to meet demand.
  - Finally, such an arrangement would speed up access to vaccines when they are developed, and would ensure long-term sustainable and affordable supply.

Drug development depends on both public and private investment

Bringing new drugs and vaccines to market is costly. For one drug to be approved by the Food and Drug Administration (FDA), a firm typically screens 5,000–10,000 compounds. Of these, an average of 250 compounds survive preclinical testing, only 5 are approved for clinical testing, and only 1 succeeds in obtaining FDA approval.[2]

Most of the R&D costs are concentrated in the clinical testing phases, and during the start-up of the manufacturing process. About 70% of R&D costs for a typical new medicine are incurred after clinical testing begins.[3] Clinical trials for vaccines tend to be larger, and thus more expensive, than those for drugs, so the proportion of costs for clinical testing is likely to be even higher.

For R&D on health conditions that affect affluent countries, a large share of the basic scientific research is funded by the public sector, while the greater part of clinical testing and drug development is financed by private sector investments. Of the total investments in health R&D across the world (about $106 billion in 2001), governments provided about 44% of the total, the pharmaceutical industry about 48% and private, nonprofit and university funds provided the remaining 8%.[4, 5]

Public and philanthropic programs in industrialized countries are focused mainly on basic research

About half of total global government funding for health research is financed by the U.S. government. U.S. funding is channeled mainly through the National Institutes of Health (NIH), part of the U.S. Department of Health and Human Services. NIH invests more than $28 billion a year, with about 80% awarded to more than 200,000 researchers in universities, medical schools and other research institutions in the United States and around the world. About 10% of the NIH budget supports projects conducted by nearly 6,000 scientists in its own laboratories.

A study of 21 drugs introduced between 1965 and 1992 and considered to have the highest therapeutic value found that public funding was instrumental in the development of 15 of them.[6] NIH notes that the work that it funds is basic research, requiring extensive further development, and that development and production of an FDA-approved therapeutic drug occurs, on average, 8–12 years after the basic research has been completed.[7]

The private nonprofit sector, including foundations, charities and universities, provided approximately $8 billion in 2002, about 8% of total global health R&D.

Public investments are complemented by commercial private investments, when the promise of a market exists. Global investment in health R&D by the for-profit sector was estimated at more than $50 billion in 2002, of which the U.S. pharmaceutical industry comprised about half. The trade association, PhRMA, estimates that the U.S. industry spent $34.4 billion on R&D in 2003.[8] However, definitions of R&D vary so this figure should simply be regarded as confirming the orders of magnitude, but not necessarily comparable to the overall figures.

Private investment in health R&D is spent primarily on developing products and turning promising candidates into drugs. A study by the National Science Foundation found that 18% of the U.S. pharmaceutical industry's spending on R&D is devoted to basic research; the other 82% toward applied research and product development.[9] Other observers estimate that about 10% of industry investment is in basic research.[10] The trade association puts the figure higher, which may again reflect differences in definition.

It is difficult to overstate the importance of private sector investment in medicines. As well as providing the majority of the investment, the incentives are particularly effective at ensuring that research is targeted at the strategies that will bring the best possible products to market as quickly as possible. Decisions about where to allocate resources are made by those with the most at stake and the most direct knowledge of the prospects of scientific success, and investment decisions are based on a hard-headed analysis without political or bureaucratic influence.

R&D funding for products for the developing world

This picture of complementary private and public investment is quite different for R&D on products for primary use in the developing world. Overall, only a tiny proportion of total R&D addresses poor country health problems—about $6 billion of a total of more than $100 billion annually; of that, less than $1 billion is devoted to vaccine research. The funding mechanisms also are markedly different: under current arrangements, progress toward drugs and vaccines for these diseases depends on public and philanthropic funding, largely through grants—with about $1 billion from philanthropic sources and $5 billion from the public sector. Very little is invested by commercial firms themselves in products specific to health problems of developing countries—which is unsurprising given the small potential returns and the high risks associated with developing country markets.

The total resources committed to developing vaccines against the three biggest global infectious diseases (HIV/AIDS, tuberculosis and malaria) is less than $1 billion a year, compared with about $100 billion spent on diseases of rich countries. This disparity is reflected in the number and type of drugs that make it to market: among 1,223 new chemical entities brought to market from 1975 to 1997, only 13 (1%) were specifically for tropical diseases; of these, only 4 were the direct results of research and development activities of the pharmaceutical industry targeted at new human products.[11]

Both empirical evidence and theory tell us that commercial investment in R&D is strongly influenced by the size of the expected market. In one study an increase of 1% in the potential market size for a drug category led to a 4–6% increase in the number of new drugs in that category.[12]

Despite the lack of commercial incentives, some pharmaceutical companies are investing in the development of vaccines to prevent rotavirus, malaria, HIV and the forms of pneumococcus prevalent in many poor countries. But these efforts, while very welcome, are modest relative to the size of problem and the amount of investment needed. To accelerate progress toward these vaccines, it is necessary to move beyond investments motivated primarily by corporate social responsibility, toward a model in which these investments can become part of the mainstream commercial business, driven by the same incentives and commercial imperatives as products for affluent markets.

Product development partnerships

A large share of R&D philanthropic spending since the mid-1990s has been channeled through about 20 product development public-private partnerships (PDPPPs), which were established to provide direct support for basic research and clinical trials in particular disease areas. Both the Rockefeller Foundation and the Bill & Melinda Gates Foundation have been instrumental in the development of the PDPPP concept and its implementation. While ad hoc collaboration between pharmaceutical companies and public sector bodies had previously existed around individual candidate projects, there were no systematic attempts to promote

the parallel development of a portfolio of candidate products—as the PDPPPs now attempt to do. Some PDPPPs are relatively new, with small portfolios; the older ones, with seven or more years' experience, manage sizeable portfolios, in some cases more than 25 products (box 2.1).

For vaccines, the main PDPPPs include the Malaria Vaccine Initiative (MVI), the International AIDS Vaccine Initiative (IAVI) and the Aeras Global TB Fund (Aeras). The majority of the funding for PDPPPs comes from philanthropic foundations—again, the Bill & Melinda Gates Foundation is the biggest contributor.

MVI, founded in 1999, has spent more than $43 million on malaria vaccine R&D and now supports 20 vaccine candidates in various stages of preclinical or clinical development. This is about 15% of total noncommercial malaria vaccine R&D expenditures from 1999 to 2003. NIH (specifically, the National Institute of Allergy and Infectious Diseases, or NIAID) accounts

---

Box 2.1
Examples of product development public-private partnerships

HIV/AIDS
- International AIDS Vaccine Initiative (IAVI)
- South African AIDS Vaccine Initiative (SAAVI)
- Global Microbicide Project (GMP)
- International Partnership for Microbicides (IPM)
- Microbicide Development Project (MDP)

Malaria
- Medicines for Malaria Venture (MMV)
- Malaria Vaccine Initiative (MVI)
- European Malaria Vaccine Initiative (EMVI)

Tuberculosis
- Global Alliance for Tuberculosis Drug Development
- Aeras Global TB Vaccine Foundation
- Foundation for Innovative New Diagnostics

Other
- Drugs for Neglected Diseases Initiative (DNDi)
- Institute for OneWorld Health (IOWH)
- Pediatric Dengue Vaccine Initiative (PDVI)
- Human Hookworm Vaccine Initiative (HHVI)

for more than 50% of total funding; other funders include the European Community, the World Health Organization's (WHO) Special Programme for Research and Training in Tropical Diseases (TDR), the U.S. Agency for International Development (USAID) and the U.S. Department of Defense.[13] MVI works through targeted partnerships with scientists, vaccinologists and development projects, and seeks to link government, industry and academic partners with field trial sites in malaria-endemic countries as early as feasible in the development process. Increasingly, MVI is recognizing the importance of working during the R&D phase to support the development of financing and introduction strategies.

A slightly different model has been used by IAVI, which was founded in 1996. IAVI is focused mainly on providing financial and technical support for product development—according to IAVI's strategic plan, it will use 75% of its budget ($340 million donated to date) to support promising vaccine candidates. IAVI currently has 20 preclinical vaccines, 5 Phase I vaccines and 1 Phase II vaccine in its portfolio.[14]

The Aeras Global TB Foundation received a grant of $82.9 million from the Bill & Melinda Gates Foundation in February 2004 to support research of promising tuberculosis vaccines in three main areas: clinical trials of two promising vaccine candidates, improving the effectiveness of animal models to indicate efficacy in humans and basic research on early-stage "next generation" candidates.[15]

These and other PDPPPs are not resourced to take a portfolio of vaccine candidates through late stage clinical trials and commercial development. Even to meet their existing mandate—that is, not including commercial product development—they are estimated to need an additional $1–2 billion over the coming two to three years.[16]

The roles of public and private investment: the malaria example

Despite the best efforts by PDPPPs, the small volume of resources for R&D and the absence of dynamic commercial investment have serious negative consequences for progress toward good—and then better—products for the world's most serious health conditions.

Consider R&D for a malaria vaccine. Total global funding of R&D for a malaria vaccine in recent years has been about $65 million annually; in addition to this, MVI recently received a $100 million grant from the Bill & Melinda Gates Foundation. This funding has enabled several candidate vaccines to move from the lab to clinical trials. So far, the scientific results are promising.

This level of funding—remarkably generous in comparison with what was previously available—represents only a fraction of the likely costs of getting a product to market. The lowest estimates of the costs of pharmaceutical development predict a total of at least $300 million per new medicine; the most widely used estimate is $802 million (in 2000 dollars).[17] Even at the lower estimates, pursuing a single candidate vaccine through the remaining phases of clinical trials, regulatory approval and production would exceed the total public and philanthropic funds presently available for the development of a malaria vaccine.

Using any plausible scenario for public and philanthropic financing alone, the available funds might allow at most one candidate to be pursued through large trials to licensure. If MVI has to bet all its available funding on a single candidate, this would eliminate its ability to fund other prospects. So there would be no fallback if the lead candidate does not succeed—or has unforeseen adverse effects. There would be no competitive pressure to improve the efficacy or reduce costs, and no prospect of second-generation products following behind.[18]

Even if funding were increased to allow a limited set of clinical trials, and if these trials demonstrate high levels of safety and efficacy, there are no guarantees that the product would be commercialized or produced in sufficient volume to support rapid uptake. The lead time for development of significant manufacturing capacity, which is beyond the scope of any public or philanthropic program, can be up to six years, and this investment is very costly and risky. "Right now, the markets don't justify the risk, from a pharmaceutical company's perspective," according to Melinda Moree, Director of Malaria Vaccine Initiative, PATH. "We have to find ways to make this work for both the private and public sector. If the market is not there, the products won't be there. Getting the incentives right could make the difference."

With the right market incentives, pharmaceutical companies have the experience, cost advantage and structure that would enable them to test and develop scientific leads and progress them as rapidly as possible through the development pipeline.

An effective vaccine against malaria would be of enormous social value. Malaria is one of the world's biggest killers of children, and through the Expanded Programme on Immunization (EPI) we have a proven and effective mechanism to deliver vaccines to children. But as things stand, the likely revenues to industry from developing a vaccine remain small. Governments in Sub-Saharan Africa cannot afford large increases in health spending. While donors might be willing to pay for life-saving products, at least for a time, a rational firm would discount that market heavily because of the downward pressure that donors collectively place on pharmaceutical prices.

Possible incentives for commercial investment

To understand better the potential for altering the behavior of pharmaceutical firms through the use of targeted incentives, we looked at several examples of how policies have affected private sector R&D activities: the U.S. Orphan Drug Act, procurement of meningitis C vaccine in the United Kingdom, incentives generated by government procurement guidelines, the Bioshield legislation in the United States and increasing the financing for existing products, with enhanced forecasting of demand.

U.S. Orphan Drug Act

The U.S. Orphan Drug Act of 1983 uses market exclusivity and other mechanisms to enhance the market and thereby stimulate R&D on products for diseases that are rare in the United States (defined as those that afflict fewer than 200,000 Americans).[19]

The Orphan Drug Act provides the following incentives:

- Seven years' marketing exclusivity on FDA approval (the FDA cannot approve the "same" drug for the same orphan indication without the sponsor's consent for seven years). If a drug demonstrates clinical superiority, the new drug can then be authorized for the same orphan disease.
- Tax credit for related clinical research, up to 50% of clinical testing expenses.
- Grant support for investigation of rare disease treatment.

The act has increased R&D. According to the FDA, more than 200 drugs and biological products for rare diseases have been brought to market since 1983, up from fewer than 10 in the previous decade.[20] Of these, only 8 preventive vaccines have been designated. The main feature that makes the act attractive to pharmaceutical companies is believed to be the promise of a period of market exclusivity.[21]

Advance contracts for meningitis C vaccine in the United Kingdom

The establishment of a more certain and commercially attractive market in the United Kingdom stimulated the development of a meningitis C vaccine.

In 1994 officials in the U.K. Department of Health noticed an increase in the notifications and laboratory-confirmed cases of meningococcal disease. While some of the increase was the result of improvements in reporting, there had also been a disproportionate increase in group C cases, particularly for older teenagers. The department conducted talks with all major pharmaceutical manufacturers to understand the status of research on a vaccine for meningitis C. These talks revealed that a product was in the early stages of development.

In 1996 the United Kingdom announced that a tender would be issued for a meningitis conjugate vaccine, and a tender for 18 million doses of vaccine was duly issued in 1999. Three companies responded to the tender and negotiations were conducted with each company separately. Clinical trial support and help by way of expedited regulatory reviews shortened the time to market for the companies in the United Kingdom and through the mutual recognition process in other European countries. The guaranteed purchase was negotiated with each company participating in the tender; the first to market would receive the lion's share of the purchase.

The first vaccine was licensed in October 1999 by Wyeth Lederle, which received a contract for approximately 10 million doses. This was followed by contracts for Chiron (5 million doses) and Baxter (3 million doses) in March and July 2000. The price was about $21 a dose. In subsequent tenders, in which only the annual birth cohort was vaccinated (approximately 240,000 births at three doses per infant), prices fell substantially and fluctuated at around $12–18 a dose. The combination of accelerated approval and guaranteed purchase brought forward the development of a conjugate meningococcal vaccine.[22]

Incentives generated by government procurement guidelines

Vaccines for Children (VFC), a U.S. government program established in 1994, provides vaccines to needy children free of charge. The Advisory Committee on Immunization Practices (ACIP), experts selected by the Department of Health and Human Services, makes recommendations on vaccines to be administered in the United States. In practice, the recommendations typically set policy for immunization requirements and determine which vaccines will be available under VFC. Hence, if a vaccine is recommended by ACIP, producers of that vaccine are assured a reasonably large market. Vaccine prices are typically negotiated after the ACIP recommendation, so once it has issued a recommendation, a vaccine producer is in a strong position to set the price close to the vaccine's social value. In this way the ACIP system shares some of the characteristics of an advance market commitment.

Similarly, the private response to the 1993 Medicare policy to cover influenza vaccinations without co-payments or deductibles, which substantially enlarged the expected market for flu vaccines, offers evidence that policies can induce R&D in the private sector.[23] The best flu vaccines in existence at the time the policy was put in place had an efficacy rate of 58%, and the 1993 flu policy helped stimulate the research responsible for the approval (in 2003) of the first new flu vaccines since 1978, as well as the first intranasal flu vaccine, FluMist, which has an 85% efficacy rate in healthy adults. The annual potential benefits from the 1993 flu policy (in particular, the combination of greater efficacy and wider use of the new vaccine) were estimated to range from $4.3–9.5 billion.[24]

Project Bioshield I and II

Project Bioshield legislation uses market enhancement mechanisms to stimulate development of bioterror countermeasures for 57 diagnostics, vaccines and therapeutic products prioritized by the Defense Science Board in the United States. Enacted in 2003, Bioshield provided for:

- Spending authority of nearly $6 billion for the procurement of qualifying countermeasures available in five years.[25]
- Greater authority of NIH and NIAID to award R&D grants and contracts and to hire technical experts.
- FDA emergency-use authorization—for example, to waive licensing requirements if a product is needed in an emergency where alternatives are not available.

A feature of the original design of Project Bioshield is that it established spending authority generally without committing to a particular price for the product. This reduces the certainty of returns to the producer: once a product has been developed,

the U.S. government would still have an incentive to bargain for a low price. Moreover, the budgetary authority expires after five years, even though it is likely to take longer to develop new products. Accordingly, the reaction of industry has been mixed. In interviews with pharmaceutical and biotech companies the Working Group found support for the need for explicit market creation, but also a widespread feeling that the proposals in the legislation had not gone far enough to achieve this

Congress is now considering a further piece of legislation, Project Bioshield II, to create incentives to encourage research including in infectious diseases, which could include tax credits, intellectual property incentives, "wild card" patents (allowing companies to recover their R&D costs by extending the patent on a different product) and liability protection

Enhancing incentives by demonstrating demand

One way to increase firms' assessment of the likely returns on investment in future products is to buy larger quantities of products that are available today. The existence of GAVI and the Vaccine Fund, which have pledges in excess of $1.3 billion for the purchase and delivery of existing vaccines, may encourage some manufacturers to look again at developing-country markets. The International Federation of Pharmaceutical Manufacturers and Associations (IFPMA) has said, "This global initiative...has led to significant improvements in financing higher levels of immunization in developing countries, making the development of new vaccines for developing countries feasible."[26]

Options for financing R&D for neglected diseases of developing countries

The question of how to provide incentives for R&D on developing-country drugs and vaccines has intrigued economists, public-policy specialists, public health experts and others for a long time, and has taken on an increasing intensity in the debates about the best way to use donor resources in the fight against AIDS, tuberculosis and malaria.

Table 2.1 provides a thumbnail sketch of various approaches that have been suggested, along with their advantages and risks. Of the "pull" proposals, an advance market commitment has the advantage that it simultaneously meets the goals of creating effective incentives for commercial investment in R&D, ensuring

Table 2.1
Possible incentives for commercial investment

Approach	Description	Advantages	Risks and challenges
Advance market commitment	Sponsor promises to fully or partially fund purchases of vaccines meeting specified conditions.	• Creates link between product quality and the revenues that accrue to a developer. • Creates market for improved vaccines and progress. • Ensures access to new vaccines in both the short and long run. • Requires sponsors to pay only if a desired product is developed.	• Promises must be credible. • Must be designed to cover appropriate products. • Requires explicit financial commitment.
Patent buyouts	Sponsor offers to buy patent rights to a vaccine meeting specified conditions, then puts the patent in the public domain and encourages competition in manufacturing the vaccine.	• Allows competition among manufacturers. • May reduce prices and thus increase access.	• Promises must be credible. • Must be designed to cover appropriate products. • Manufacturer may have effective monopoly. • Uncertain link between payments and product quality. • Likely to be winner-takes-all.
Strengthened intellectual property right (IPR) protection	Public sector makes stronger commitment to enforce or extend IPRs (similar to Orphan Drug Act's guaranteed market exclusivity).	• Provides some additional incentive for industry.	• Difficult to implement. • Higher prices for longer will impede access. • May be politically unpopular. • Provides very little incentive for R&D on products specific to poor countries.
Sales tax credits	Government offers a tax credit on vaccine sales.	• Provides some additional incentive for industry to invest.	• Only of benefit to those with a tax liability (unless credits are transferable). • Must be credible; no recourse to legal challenge for changes in tax law. • Difficult to coordinate internationally.
Prizes	Offers cash or other reward to whoever achieves a certain, pre-specified goal.	• Provides immediate upfront payment—no need for long-term contract.	• Industry may not be enthusiastic about competing for prizes. • Does not address access. • Winner takes all. • Does not foster competition for subsequent improvements.

Promoting private investment in vaccine development

(continued on next page)

2

Table 2.1 (continued)
Possible incentives for commercial investment

Approach	Description	Advantages	Risks and challenges
Prizes based on incremental benefits[a]	Innovators are rewarded based on the incremental therapeutic benefits; plus compulsory licensing.	• Solves access problem. • Reduces wasteful duplication. • Applies to wide range of diseases.	• Difficulty of fairly determining social value after products have been developed. • May be insufficient to foster competition for subsequent innovation. • Uncertainty of value may deter investment.
Best entry tournaments	Offers cash or other reward to whoever progresses farthest toward a specific research goal by a given date.	• Provides assurance that reward will be paid.	• May have to pay without getting result. • Does not address access.
Patent extensions on existing pharmaceuticals ("wildcard patents")	Gives a manufacturer the right to extend the patent on any product in an industrial market, or allows a manufacturer to extend the customary time period that a patent is protected.	• Is attractive to larger pharmaceutical companies.	• Favors big companies and those with existing patents (unless patent extensions are transferable). • Places cost of developing new vaccines on users of drugs whose patent is extended. • Winner takes all—does not foster competition for subsequent improvements.
R&D treaty[b]	An international R&D treaty under which each signatory promises to devote a minimum fraction of its GDP to drug research through diverse mechanisms.	• Spreads R&D costs internationally. • Is consistent with different intellectual property regimes.	• Free-rider problem: individual countries may channel subsidies to within-country firms and universities rather than to fund R&D on usable products suitable for poor countries. • Does not directly address access.
Virtual pharma	A drug development strategy in which a small management team acquires and monitors most of its R&D services from outside vendors.	• Coordinates research. • Prevents unnecessary duplication. • Encourages information sharing.	• Lack of competition for innovation. • Funders may not be best-placed to choose which research strategies to pursue. • Absence of strong managerial incentives may lead to bureaucracy. • Does not take advantage of R&D cost advantage of pharmaceutical industry. • Uncertainty of future funding.

Table 2.1 (continued)
Possible incentives for commercial investment

Approach	Description	Advantages	Risks and challenges
Limiting patent protection in poor countries[c]	Allowing patent protection in rich markets coupled with unrestricted competition by generics manufacturers in poor countries.	• Ensures increased access with little loss to pharmaceutical industry. • Is cheap to implement.	• Is not intended to address problem of neglected diseases, but rather on medicines for which markets exist in high-income countries.
Fast-track regulatory approval	Rewarding pharmaceutical companies for developing vaccines for low-income countries by fast-tracking regulatory approval for them or for other, more profitable medicines.	• Benefits to pharmaceutical companies at little cost. • Complements other approaches.	• Reward insufficiently large and insufficiently certain. • If regulatory approval is being unnecessarily delayed, it should be accelerated anyway.

Note: This table draws on Glass, Batson and Levine (2001) and Kremer and Glennerster (2004), with additions.

a. Hollis (2005).

b. Hubbard and Love (2004).

c. Lanjouw (2003).

funding for rapid and affordable access to vaccines once they are developed and creating incentives for competition among suppliers and for further development of improved second-generation products. It is this approach that the Center for Global Development's Advance Market Commitment Working Group examined in detail.

The potential benefits of an advance market commitment

An advance market commitment, in which suppliers of vaccines that meet established technical specifications are guaranteed a price that provides the potential for a viable return on investment, closely mimics for the developing world the type of market incentives that exist in the developed world. In principle, such an arrangement could have important benefits:

• It would mobilize additional resources, particularly for the clinical testing phases of development. Despite generous funding by foundations, within current budget envelopes most of the product development public-private partnerships and other "push" programs that are engaged in drug and vaccine development for the developing world do not have sufficient resources to bring products through the full R&D process. As noted earlier in the case of malaria, without significant commercial investment it is not clear how multiple candidate vaccines will be moved through clinical testing and, potentially, into large-scale manufacture.

• It would engage the dynamism and energy of the commercial pharmaceutical sector—from biotechs to multinational firms. It would mean that decisions about which avenues to pursue, and which to abandon, would be put in the hands of those with the biggest stake and with the most knowledge about the prospects for success. It would harness the incentives and managerial capacity of the industry to develop new vaccines rapidly. It would thereby reproduce for developing-country diseases the market-based incentives that, together with public and philanthropic funding of R&D, have contributed to tremendous innovation in medicines for affluent countries, rewarding firms that move fastest toward the objective of developing and producing good products.

- It allows public sector and philanthropic funders to stand at arm's length from complex scientific choices and tradeoffs, avoiding the need for them to take a position on the feasible approaches and the likelihood of success. By clearly defining the objectives they wish to achieve with public funds, the sponsors can create conditions in which a variety of different approaches can be tried, not all of which may command a scientific consensus at the outset, promote competition and allow different firms to make their own judgments about the scientific feasibility and risks of alternative strategies.

- It would pay for results, providing sponsors with the assurance that large-scale funding would be provided if and only if an effective and safe product that is appropriate for the developing world is manufactured in large enough quantity to meet demand. This is consistent with innovations in development assistance, in which donors seek to pay for results rather than inputs.

- It would make the most of the untapped asset of information. By informing potential developers and suppliers about how much they would be willing to pay, and then locking it in, donors provide the type of signal that can, quite literally, be turned into capital.

- Properly designed, it would ensure access by helping to purchase vaccines in the short run and by ensuring a sustainable supply at an affordable price in the long run

There is widespread agreement that more must be done to accelerate progress toward new vaccines and other products for the developing world. Similarly, there is broad appreciation of the value of engaging the talent, resources and hard-nosed business sense of the private sector in developing and pursuing promising scientific pathways, and creating efficient manufacturing processes. From a conceptual perspective, providing an advance market commitment is appealing: it builds on the best aspects of markets, deploying public resources responsibly to stimulate private innovation.

But could it work? Would it work? What would be the potential costs and benefits? The findings of the Working Group on these questions are presented in the chapters that follow.

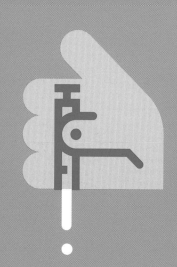

3
A market
not a prize

Chapter at a glance

- The idea of making an advance purchase commitment has been discussed for several years, but the details of how it could be implemented have not been worked out. Our Working Group was established to determine whether a commitment could be designed that could be implemented and that would be effective and good value for money.
- We propose a framework for an advance market commitment that would bring new impetus to R&D in vaccines for diseases occurring mainly in developing countries. The arrangements are intended to create a market analogous to the market for medicines in affluent countries.
- Our proposal is for a market not a prize. There is no winner-take-all.

By underwriting the purchase of vaccines, donors create incentives for firms to compete to bring products to market quickly. Better products can compete for market share, as they can in affluent markets.

- Advance market commitments would accelerate the production and availability of late stage products (rotavirus and pneumococcus vaccines) as well as the R&D and availability of early stage products (vaccines for malaria, HIV, tuberculosis).
- We have set out a quantified example for a malaria vaccine. A market worth $3 billion would create incentives for commercial investment to accelerate R&D, and the purchase of the vaccines at $15 per dose for the first

200 million people would provide remarkable value for money for donors—less than $15 per life-year saved.

- The commitment has been designed to meet the needs of all stakeholders. It would be of significant benefit to donors, industry and most of all the people in developing countries.
- An advance market commitment would fill an important gap in our arrangements for R&D for global health challenges. But our enthusiasm for it does not diminish the importance we attach to a range of other measures that we can and should take in the near term to save lives immediately and to enhance the prospect of developing new medicines that are essential for developing countries.

A practical advance market commitment

We have developed a new proposal for an advance market commitment that responds to the needs of donors, industry and the public health community. Unlike some alternative "pull" proposals, as summarized in chapter 2, this commitment does not create a prize to reward R&D.[1] Instead it creates a market, broadly reproducing the market incentives to develop medicines for affluent countries (box 3.1).

We worked with experts in public policy, law, economics, health and scientific research, and we consulted potential sponsors and firms in the pharmaceutical and biotech sectors, in developed countries

---

Box 3.1
The main features of the commitment

- A technical specification—in terms of outputs—required of a new vaccine.
- A minimum price guarantee, available up to a fixed number of treatments.
- Guaranteed co-payments on products meeting the specification, paid by sponsors, permitting eligible countries to buy vaccines at affordable prices, for a maximum number of treatments. (For example, the price might be fixed at $15 per treatment, with the developing country perhaps paying $1 and the sponsors paying $14, for up to 200 million treatments).
- An overall market size of about $3 billion—enough to make it worthwhile for firms with scientific opportunities to undertake research and development, but well below the social value of the vaccine.
- An independent adjudication committee to oversee the arrangements and commitments enforceable under the law.
- An obligation on the producer to produce and sell further treatments in eligible countries at a fixed, affordable price, in return for having had the advantage of sales at the initial higher price.
- Total sales of each qualifying product would depend on demand from developing countries. This in turn would depend on the effectiveness of the vaccine and the alternatives available.

---

and in India. Our aim has been to determine whether it would be possible, in practice, for sponsors to make a commitment that would be effective in accelerating the development of new vaccines.

The advance market commitment proposed here aims to mimic the size and certainty of a market for medicines in affluent countries, and so create similar incentives for commercial investment in R&D. As well as accelerating the development of new vaccines, this approach would create incentives for rapid, large-scale production and provide the funds needed to buy the vaccines when they are available.

We conclude that an advance market commitment is indeed practical and that it would be effective. This chapter outlines the main features of how a commitment could work, summarizing the implications for the main stakeholders. The rest of the report considers the design of the commitment and its likely impact in more detail.

Commitments for late-stage and early-stage products

The idea of an advance market commitment is this: because the potential market is made more valuable and more certain, firms will make investment decisions that accelerate the development of products for developing countries and invest in manufacturing capacity to produce larger volumes. This analysis applies both to late-stage products (those in the final stages of regulatory approval and for which manufacturing capacity is being established, such as rotavirus vaccine) and to early-stage products (those requiring scientific progress and extensive testing of candidate medicines, such as malaria or HIV vaccines).

The impact of an advance market commitment for late-stage products

The rationale for using an advance market commitment for late-stage products is that, even after a product has proven successful in clinical trials, the low and uncertain value of demand from developing countries continues to affect the firm's investment decisions, which will determine the speed, volume and price of making the vaccine available.

The firm's decisions that will be affected by market prospects include:

- Whether and how quickly to conduct clinical trials in developing countries.[2]

- Whether to make a version of the product with the specification and presentation suitable for developing countries.
- The speed of obtaining regulatory approval for developing countries.
- Whether enough production capacity is put in place for large-volume, low-unit-cost production.
- The price of the product in developing countries.

Each of these decisions is critically affected by the prospects for future demand from developing countries, by the predictability of that demand and by the price the firm expects for sales to those markets. Experience has shown that, in the absence of reliable demand for developing-country markets, firms prefer to focus first on producing new vaccines in low volumes and selling them mainly into high-value, developed-country markets. When high-value market needs have been met, and as the competition from lower cost generics producers becomes more likely, producers move toward the high-volume, low-cost production needed for the developing world.

Using an advance market commitment for late-stage products would:

- Accelerate the availability of new vaccines in large quantities and at low prices, adapted as necessary for use in developing countries, creating a virtuous circle (figure 3.1).

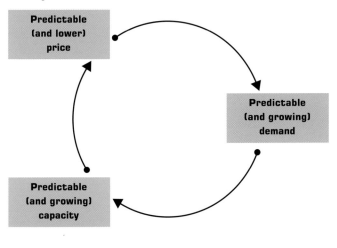

Figure 3.1
A virtuous circle of demand, capacity and price

- Accelerate uptake of new vaccines by guaranteeing an affordable long-term price once the commitment is exhausted.
- Ensure affordable access for people who need vaccines.
- Add to the credibility of the commitment for early-stage products and so accelerate the development of new vaccines.

The impact of an advance market commitment for early-stage products

Firms cannot make substantial investments in R&D if the market for the final product is expected to be small and risky. The pharmaceutical industry has to decide where to invest its resources based on its expectation of success and its estimate of the value of the market. As long as the market for vaccines for developing countries remains small, there is little incentive for commercial investment in vaccines for diseases concentrated in developing countries.

The case for an advance market commitment for early-stage products is that it would create an expected return from developing-country markets large enough for some pharmaceutical firms to increase their investment in R&D in these products.

In practice, pharmaceutical companies invest in R&D through a combination of work in their own laboratories, contract research, licensing intellectual property from others and acquiring or entering joint ventures with other pharmaceutical and biotech companies. These investments are made by the company on the basis of the long-term expected returns from market sales of a new product. Both empirical evidence and theory tell us that commercial investment in R&D is strongly influenced by the size of the expected market. In one study an increase of 1% in the potential market size for a drug category led to a 4–6% increase in the number of new drugs in that category.[3]

If an advance market commitment creates incentives for pharmaceutical companies to invest in R&D, those companies will in turn create a range of more immediate incentives within the R&D community. The market value of discoveries relating to global health issues will rise. More research contracts will be signed. Venture capitalists will increase investment in biotechs. In this way, the incentive created by the establishment of a final market will "reach back" to create more immediate incentives for the intermediate research outputs required. Biotech companies and their investors will not have to invest on the basis of returns that are likely to take 10 or more years to materialize. If they are successful, they can expect to license their products to pharmaceutical companies much faster than that. The basis for our expectation that this will work in practice is that this is precisely how collaboration on R&D on products for affluent markets works. There may be room for improvement in the way these contracts are created. But the functioning of these markets gives us good reason to believe that a healthy market for intermediate outputs would follow from a suitable advance market commitment for the end product.

In addition to creating incentives for R&D, an early-stage advance market commitment would have the same benefits as a late-stage advance market commitment in that it would create incentives for high-volume, low-unit-cost production and ensure financing for access to these vaccines.

Design differences between early-stage and late-stage commitments

The main difference between the design of an early-stage commitment and a late-stage commitment is that the contract for late-stage products would likely be with specific named suppliers while the contract for early-stage products would initially be an open framework agreement, with firms competing for the right to benefit from the guaranteed price in the second contract.

We set out below examples of how an advance market commitment could work for malaria (an early-stage product) and pneumococcus or rotavirus (late-stage products). These examples were developed to focus and discipline the thinking of the Working Group. They do not necessarily imply that these should be the diseases for which a commitment would be most appropriate.

A sample advance market commitment for malaria

We looked at malaria as an example of a specific case where advance contracting is needed to complement ongoing public and philanthropic funding efforts to accelerate development of an essential early-stage vaccine. We are particularly grateful to the staff of the Malaria Vaccine Initiative for contributions to this analysis, though they are not responsible for the analyses or the conclusions.

The need for advance contracting for malaria

The World Health Organization estimates that at least 2.3 billion people are at risk from malaria and at least 1 million people, possibly as many as 2 million, die of the disease each year.[4] It is possible that estimates of the burden of diseases will be increased during 2005 as a result of new analysis.

More than half of all malaria deaths are among children in Sub-Saharan Africa. Though estimates of economic impact are necessarily based on imperfect information and multiple assumptions, some studies have estimated that malaria may reduce average economic growth in Africa by half a percentage point a year or more.[5]

Malaria transmission occurs through the bite of an infected anopheles mosquito. Parasites multiply in the liver and red blood cells of affected people. Symptoms include fever, headache, muscular aches and weakness, vomiting and diarrhea. The disease may result in long-term debilitation or be fatal if untreated or treated with ineffective drugs.

Malaria was almost completely eradicated from North American and Europe using insecticides and environmental management. But the same can not be achieved elsewhere, for a combination of climatic and biological reasons. Africa's temperatures, mosquito species and humidity give the continent the highest malaria burden. Africa's malaria mosquitoes almost exclusively bite humans, which enhances the chain of human-to-human transmission. The combination of high temperatures, sufficient rainfall for mosquito breeding and human-biting anopheles mosquitoes make it much more difficult to control the disease than elsewhere. In addition, there is increasingly widespread resistance to malaria drugs and insecticides. Given that childhood vaccinations already reach more than 75% of the world's children, and the immense challenge of controlling the mosquito vector, an effective malaria vaccine suitable for young children, which could be delivered through the EPI schedule, and for women of childbearing age would be a major and much needed addition to the prevention strategies such as insecticide-treated bednets and vector control.

In addition to public funding through organizations such as NIH, two initiatives provide "push" support for malaria vaccines:

- The European Malaria Vaccine Initiative, founded in 1998 by the European Union, provides a mechanism to facilitate the development of candidate molecules through the post-validation phase of nationally and internationally funded malaria vaccine R&D—and to see candidate molecules through to limited clinical trials in close collaboration with the African Malaria Network Trust. This is intended to ensure that appropriate vaccines are developed as quickly as possible.

- The Malaria Vaccine Initiative (MVI) was founded at the Program for Appropriate Technology in Health in 1999 with funding from the Bill & Melinda Gates Foundation. It has received total funding to date of $150 million. Of the 20 vaccine candidates MVI is supporting, 8 have entered clinical development (Phase I or Phase II clinical trials).

Malaria vaccine research has made painstaking gains over many years. With its multistage life cycle, malaria presents a unique and complex vaccine challenge. There are no vaccines on the market, but three types of vaccines are in development, targeting points in the malaria life cycle: pre-erythrocytic, blood stage and transmission stage.

In October 2004 researchers reported preliminary results from the largest vaccine efficacy trial ever conducted in Africa.[6] This Phase II trial in Mozambique of a vaccine[7] was supported by MVI and GSK Biologicals. The trial found vaccine efficacy of 30% against clinical malaria attacks, 45% against primary infection with *Plasmodium falciparum* and 58% against severe disease. Further progress on this candidate vaccine will depend, however, on there being sufficient investment. There may be other candidate vaccines that would be as effective or more so but for which there are not sufficient resources to conduct trials.

While collaboration between philanthropic foundations and the private sector has had a significant impact on malaria vaccine development, a complementary mechanism to enhance the market is also needed for at least two reasons, as noted in chapter 2. First, more research is needed in a wider range of candidate vaccines to identify the best opportunities and accelerate progress on those ideas. Experts are in broad agreement that the first malaria vaccine will be only partially efficacious, and efforts will be required to develop superior products as new knowledge about the immune response is obtained. The most successful vaccines are likely to be second or third generation.

Second, today's funds are not sufficient to pursue enough of the possible avenues of research. After Phase II trials, the cost of developing and testing a candidate vaccine in humans escalate,

and progress toward commercialization will require the prospect of a sufficient market to make it economically viable. Even if MVI put all its funding into a single candidate, and if that proved a success, there would not be enough money to bring that one candidate to licensure, nor into full-scale production.

Proposed contract structure for malaria

The proposed structure for an advance market contract for malaria is set out in draft contract terms sheets in appendix F (the Framework Agreement) and appendix G (the Guarantee Agreement). These drafts are annotated with rationales and explanations.

The main characteristics of the commitment are as follows:

- The sponsors will make a legally binding promise to pay $14 of the cost of up to 200 million treatments purchased, at a guaranteed price of $15 per treatment (adjusted for inflation).
- Recipient countries will pay $1 per treatment. This can be subsidized by donor funding at the time.
- In return, firms will guarantee to provide further treatments (after the 200 million) at a sustainable base price, reflecting the cost of production, about $1 per treatment.
- An Independent Adjudication Committee will be established to determine whether the technical specification of the vaccine had been met.
- If a firm develops a subsequent, superior product (as agreed by the Independent Adjudication Committee), that product will also be eligible for the price guarantee (the price guarantee would apply to the first 200 million treatments bought, shared among the eligible products according to demand).

This offer will create an expected market of some $3 billion, approximately the average revenues for which new pharmaceuticals have been developed for affluent countries (see chapter 5). A commitment of this magnitude should attract some pharmaceutical companies to invest in R&D.

It is important to remember that the figures indicated above were developed as a working example, and we are not making specific recommendations. Further work and expert consultation would be required to set such parameters, in the event that a sponsor wished to create an advance market commitment.

Under very conservative assumptions—for example, ignoring the benefits of herd immunity, and the savings from health care costs averted—we estimate that the cost will be about $15 per disability-adjusted life year (DALY) saved (discounted in 2004 dollars), making vaccine purchases under the program one of the world's most cost-effective development interventions (box 3.2 and table 3.1). Once the commitment of 200 million doses has expired, the cost of the vaccine will fall to the sustainable long-run price.

Advance market commitments for rotavirus and pneumococcus

Recent developments in a vaccine for rotavirus

Rotavirus is the most common cause of severe dehydrating diarrhea among children worldwide. Each year it causes more than 100 million cases of disease, 25 million clinic visits and between 350,000 and 590,000 deaths in children ages five or younger. Nearly every child in the world is exposed to rotavirus before reaching age five, but, because of lack of access to health care, the children who die of rotavirus are in the very poorest countries.

At present, the only treatment for rotavirus involves preventing dehydration by providing fluids and salts until the disease runs its course; neither antibiotics nor other drugs can cure rotavirus.

A vaccine has recently been licensed in Mexico: a human-derived, monovalent, live, attenuated two-to-three-dose oral vaccine developed by Avant Immunotherapeutics and licensed to GSK Biologicals. This product has undergone Phase III trials in Latin America and is in Phase II trials in Bangladesh, Singapore and South Africa. A second vaccine is close to licensure: a bovine-human reassortant, pentavalent, live-attenuated three-dose oral vaccine developed by Merck is now in Phase III trials in Central and South America. In addition, Biovirx has recently indicated that it will pursue licensing for a rotavirus vaccine that had previously been sold in the U.S. market but was withdrawn for fears of adverse effects.[9]

Box 3.2
What is a DALY?

A disability-adjusted life year, or DALY, is a unit used for measuring both the global burden of disease and the effectiveness of health intervention. DALYs were introduced as a unit of measurement in the World Development Report 1993: Investing in Health (World Bank 1993), and in 1996 a joint effort by WHO, the World Bank and the Harvard School of Public Health produced The Global Burden of Disease (Murray and Lopez 1996) in which the DALY methodology and findings were presented in more detail.

DALYs are intended to combine losses from premature death, defined as the differences between actual age at death and life expectancy at that age in a low-mortality population, and losses of healthy life resulting from disability. Because the benefits of all health interventions can be measured this way, DALYs allow comparisons between different interventions and overcome some of the problems associated with using analysis relevant only for specific conditions or that relies on placing a monetary value on saving lives.

Table 3.1
Some estimates of the cost per DALY of development interventions

Intervention	Cost per DALY ($)[a]
Malaria vaccine under advance market commitment of $15 per treatment (conservative estimate)	15
Condom distribution	12–99
Integrated management of childhood illness	30–100
Tuberculosis prevention	169–288
Antiretroviral therapy for HIV	1,100–1,800[b]
Family planning	20–30[c]
Prenatal and delivery care	30–50
Water supply (village pump)	94
Malaria bednets	19–85
Malaria residual spraying	16–19

a. Data not adjusted for inflation. Some interventions may have changed in price substantially since these studies.

b. The cost of antiretroviral therapy has fallen since this study.

Source: Creese and others (2002); Murray and Lopez (1996); Cairncross and Valdmanis (2004); Hanson and others (2003).

Second-generation products—at the Lanzhou Institute in China, Bharat Biotech International in India, BioFarma in Indonesia and NIH—are in progress but several years behind.

The Rotavirus ADIP was established by GAVI to lay the foundation for rapid introduction and sustainable supply of first-generation rotavirus vaccines. One of the most important elements of this project is to secure the supply of affordable vaccines in predictable quantities.

Recent developments in a vaccine for pneumococcus

More children die each year from pneumonia than from any other disease—even more than malaria or AIDS—and nearly all these deaths occur in the world's poorest countries.[10] Unlike malaria and AIDS, vaccines are available to prevent these deaths. But without a coordinated effort and forward planning, it will probably take 20 years or more for these vaccines to reach even half the children in the world's poorest countries—in part because of the high cost but also because of the lack of reliable and predictable demand.

A vaccine against the second-leading cause of bacterial pneumonia deaths—a bacterium called Hib (*Haemophilus influenzae* type B)—has been available since the late 1980s. It has been widely used in all wealthy countries, and as a result Hib disease has nearly disappeared altogether in those countries. But in 2002—15 years after the vaccine was first used in wealthy countries—fewer than 15% of the world's poorest children were receiving the vaccine.

The leading cause of bacterial pneumonia deaths—a bacterium called *Streptococcus pneumoniae* (pneumococcus)—is now preventable by immunization with a vaccine very similar to the Hib vaccine. In 2000 the United States licensed a pneumococcal conjugate vaccine for prevention of severe pneumococcal infections in infants and young children. Like the Hib conjugate vaccines, this vaccine has proven to be safe and very effective in randomized clinical trials. In studies in Finland and the United States, the vaccine was shown to significantly reduce the incidence of severe pneumococcal infections, such as meningitis, pneumonia and septicemia, and to prevent ear infections. Since 2000 it has been routinely used in the United States and other wealthy countries but not in the developed world.

GAVI's Pneumococcal ADIP aims to increase access to new life-saving pneumococcal vaccines and ultimately prevent millions of deaths by getting vaccines where they are needed most, faster than ever. The ADIP has articulated a three-part mission: to establish, communicate and deliver the value of existing (and next-generation) pneumococcal vaccines. The ADIP is currently funding disease surveillance networks, clinical trials in target populations and cost-effectiveness studies. An important part of its mission will depend on delivering products to GAVI's target countries at a price and volume that they can afford.

Goals of an advance market commitment for pneumococcus and rotavirus

Against this background, an advance market commitment will:

- Ensure that first-generation products are tested in the populations that need them most.
- Provide an incentive for suppliers to produce the vaccine in quantities that will meet the needs of the developing world over time.
- Influence decisions about the presentation and characteristics of the product so that it better meets the needs of the developing world.
- Influence the long-term pricing of the product.

There is a clear need for advance market commitments to secure the right profile, price and supply of these vaccines. Combined with more concerted demand-side interventions, this will be instrumental in shortening the gap of 10–15 years seen in the introduction of recent vaccines, such as hepatitis B and Hib vaccine. The ADIPs for pneumococcus and rotavirus are important steps in this direction and, while they do not yet have the mandate to negotiate such contracts, they consider long-term advance contracting as potentially critical to achieving their mission.

Proposed contract structure for a late-stage product

We considered an advance contract for late-stage products, which could be applied to vaccines for rotavirus and pneumococcus.

Unlike the early-stage contract, the late-stage contract in these cases will be with one or more specific suppliers. (The Framework Agreement stage included in the early stage contracts would be unnecessary.) The contract with the supplier will be very similar to the Guarantee Agreement of an early-stage product.

The main characteristics of the agreement will be as follows:

- The sponsor commits to pay a relatively high price for a course of immunization, up to a certain number (say, the first 100 million courses).
- In return for receiving the higher price at first, the supplier guarantees to provide vaccine indefinitely to qualifying countries, at a much lower price. The lower, long-run price would be set at a reasonable mark-up over the estimated production cost.
- If the supplier does not fulfill demand at this lower price, given adequate notice, the contract would provide for damages, or require that a restricted license be given to the sponsor or to the public domain (to supply only Vaccine Fund–eligible countries).
- The contract might commit the sponsor to guarantee some minimum order, but after the initial volume is reached, the vaccine may have to compete against other products, so there would still be an incentive for other firms to enter if they could produce superior products or manufacture more cheaply.
- The contract could be signed prior to regulatory approval, but it is conditional on regulatory approval and the expected performance of the vaccine.

There are a number of advantages to this approach for developing countries, for suppliers and for sponsors.

- The supplier obtains a more predictable revenue stream.
- The supplier has incentives to install capacity quickly, since the net present value of its revenue will be greater the faster the first 100 million people are immunized.
- There is no long-term commitment to buy the product if a superior product is developed later.
- Both suppliers and consumers are better off than they would be with a system of short-run contracts with a single supplier. Uncertainty will be reduced for both. If prices are chosen appropriately, overall revenue and profits will increase, making the supplier better off. But the number of immunizations will also increase significantly, lowering the average price per person immunized and improving cost-effectiveness.
- The contract ensures sustainability for countries and donors in the long run. Because countries know that they will have access to the vaccine at affordable prices over the long run, they can be more confident in adding it to their immunization

schedules without fear that they will not be able to afford the vaccine later and will have to reverse their strategy.

- The contract sets a good precedent for advance market commitments aimed at stimulating investment in early-stage products—and builds confidence in that commitment mechanism.

Risks and benefits of an advance market commitment

We have based our design of the advance market commitment on economic principles, practical realities and extensive consultation with donors, industry and the public health community. We set out here how the mechanism we have designed meets the principal objectives of the main stakeholders and the risks and challenges that the commitment must address.

Benefits for donors

- The commitment would likely accelerate the development of new vaccines, which are one of the most cost-effective ways to tackle poverty, improve the health of vulnerable populations and meet the Millennium Development Goals.
- There will be a cost to sponsors only if the program succeeds and a new vaccine is developed. If no vaccine is developed, there is no significant cost to the sponsors. If a vaccine is developed, it will save millions of lives at very low cost. The commitment is payment-for-results.[11]
- If a vaccine is developed, it will be available rapidly to people who need it, in contrast to recent experience with new vaccines.
- Vaccine purchases under the commitment will be a highly cost-effective use of aid in comparison with other interventions.
- Existing and future donor support for R&D investment will be more productive as a result of complementary private investment.
- Donors will increase the productivity of their likely future expenditure by making it predictable.
- The commitment is sustainable; once the advance market at a guaranteed price has been exhausted, the suppliers will provide further vaccines at a guaranteed low price, unlike open-ended commitments to subsidize purchases indefinitely.

- Aid spending on R&D for, and delivery of, vaccines is low risk, with few opportunities for corruption and rent-seeking.

Points for donors to watch

- It is important not to be locked into a contract to spend $3 billion on a vaccine that is not needed, for reasons unforeseen at the time the commitment is made. *The commitment to create a market, rather than a prize, protects donors by ensuring that their commitment is to underwrite the cost of vaccines for which there is actually demand.*

- The commitment should be structured in a way that does not require donors to move money from current priorities, including health R&D, so that it is available for uncertain future obligations to purchase a vaccine. *A commitment to purchase a vaccine if and when it is available does not score in public spending until the vaccine is supplied. In the meantime, existing expenditure priorities can continue to be funded (chapter 7 explains in more detail).*

- Donors should avoid unnecessarily driving up the price of vaccines. *The structure of the contract ensures that the higher prices paid for the initial doses leads more quickly to long-term sustainable prices, keeping long run costs down; by contrast, under current arrangements, increased funding of vaccine purchases is likely to push up prices. Furthermore, compared with a cost-plus arrangement, an advance market commitment creates stronger incentives to keep the costs of production as low as possible to recoup the highest profit.*

- Donors should not overpay for R&D costs of vaccine development. *We don't know for certain what it will cost to develop a new vaccine. Creating commercial incentives for competition in the most expensive phases of the process will allow firms to make judgments about the best use of available resources. A larger donor commitment will encourage more competition and faster development of a new vaccine—which would be money well spent.*

Benefits for industry

- The commitment would extend the overall size of the market in which firms operate, creating opportunities to expand the scope of their business and providing a new path for growth.

- The commitment significantly reduces the risk that, if a life-saving health product is invented, it will be subject to compulsory licensing, or that the firm will be forced to sell it at a loss, either because of pressure of public opinion or because of the purchasing power of public procurement.

- The advance market commitment creates a risk-reward structure that firms are already familiar with and that puts these decisions in the same framework as other investments: they will be rewarded if they bring a product to market that governments want to buy.

- Unlike many of the alternative proposals for increasing R&D in diseases concentrated in developing countries, the advance market commitment addresses the access issue without weakening incentives or dismantling the system of intellectual property rights.

- The opportunity for commercially driven investment in vaccines reduces the risk of growing activism and anger directed at pharmaceutical companies because of the perceived lack of investment in neglected diseases—and because of the need to charge prices that make essential medicines unaffordable to the very poor.

- The commitment does not reduce donor resources available for the purchase of existing vaccines and drugs or for the investment in health systems, which increase demand for existing products.

Points for industry to watch

- The donors must not be able to renege on their commitment when a vaccine is developed that meets the technical specification. *The advance market commitment would be legally binding and enforceable in the courts. The Independent Adjudication Committee, which decides if a vaccine qualifies for the co-payment guarantee, is an important safeguard for industry, and industry should pay close attention to its composition, funding and organizational arrangements.*

- The commitment must not allow copy products to take the guaranteed market. *The Independent Adjudication Committee is responsible for ensuring that second and subsequent products that meet the technical specification are superior, and not merely generic copies.*

- A substantial portion of demand risk remains with the firm. *The market guarantee removes the risk relating to the poverty of the final consumer and the incentives of the public purchaser to secure the best possible price once the R&D costs are sunk. The demand risks that (rightly) remain with firms relate to the quality of the product, the quality of competitors and the speed of making the product available. These are risks that firms are best placed to manage—and risks that firms are used to bearing in affluent markets. The two-stage pricing structure—with bigger returns early on—greatly reduces the risk to firms and encourages early innovation. As shown in chapter 4, even if uptake is somewhat slow, the risk to firms is still much lower than it would be with a constant price.*

- The creation of a market for the final product may not be enough to create incentives for intermediate R&D. *A market of this size, combined with the response from the pharmaceutical industry, has been enough to spur the biotech sector and venture capitalist investment in R&D for pharmaceuticals for affluent markets.*

Benefits for developing countries

- An advance market commitment is likely significantly to accelerate the development of essential vaccines, the best hope for sustainably improving the health of people in poor countries.
- The commitment ensures that, if a new vaccine is developed, it will be rapidly available in developing countries at an affordable price, unlike previous vaccines, which have been available only after a long delay.
- There are many very poor people in countries that are not currently eligible for Vaccine Fund support, for whom it is a priority to increase affordable access to vaccines. For countries that are not eligible for vaccines purchased under the advance market commitment there would still be considerable benefits arising from the advance market commitment, because significantly more new vaccines would be likely to be produced.
- Experts and decisionmakers from developing countries could participate in the initial establishment of the technical specifications, ensuring that products developed are appropriate to in-country conditions.
- The commitment offers open competition for developing-country biotechs and larger firms to compete to provide new

vaccines, perhaps through joint ventures with multinational pharmaceutical companies.

- There are no adverse macroeconomic or exchange rate effects for developing countries as a result of increased development assistance provided in the form of co-payments for imported pharmaceuticals.

Points for developing countries to watch

- The contract must allow superior products to be bought if they are developed. *Because this is a market not a prize, developing countries can switch demand to superior products that qualify for the guarantee as soon as they are available.*
- Developing countries will have to make some payments for the vaccines. *The payments will be small, because donors bear most of the guaranteed price. The developing countries' contribution ensures that they are the ultimate customers for the vaccines and can decide their priorities. As is the case today, recipient countries can seek donor assistance for their contributions when the vaccines are available.*
- The long-term price must be affordable. *The commitment ensures that vaccines will be available to all eligible countries at affordable prices in the long term (and that the higher price will be subsidized by donors in the meantime). This ensures that vaccine programs are sustainable in the long run, and so enables governments to expand their vaccination programs with confidence.*

An advance market commitment is only a partial solution

Theory and evidence predict that an advance market commitment would substantially increase commercial investment in R&D on vaccines for developing countries and that it would accelerate the development and availability of new vaccines.

But much else can and should be done to accelerate R&D and improve access to vaccines. Steps that could make a substantial contribution include:

- Greater donor funding of the purchase of existing vaccines and drugs for diseases in developing countries, which will save many lives immediately and increase the perceived value of the market in the future.

- Increased upfront donor funding of R&D into health conditions concentrated in developing countries, including investment in R&D for new vaccines.
- Improved demand forecasting to enable producers to invest in manufacturing capacity of an appropriate size.

Advance market commitments are an additional tool, focused on an important deficiency in the current arrangements for the development of new vaccines: the lack of adequate incentives for commercial investment. We consider that commercial engagement in the development of new vaccines is critical for the rapid development and production of new vaccines. We believe that advance market commitments can and will make a substantial contribution to accelerating new vaccines and that they should be a high priority for donors and the industry. But in advocating their rapid introduction we are mindful of the need not to lose sight of the importance of other steps that would also improve the effectiveness of the market for vaccines.

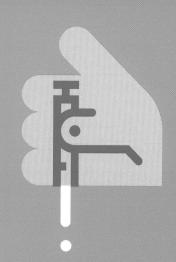

4
Design choices

Chapter at a glance

- The legal framework for an advance market commitment is founded on ordinary contract law. (See the draft contract term sheets in appendixes F and G.)
- Our multidisciplinary team comprising lawyers, public health specialists, economists and public policy specialists has considered the detailed design of the commitment with the aim of creating an appropriate set of incentives.
- We explain our recommendations for the arrangements for the structure of the contract, the technical specification of the vaccine and the organization of the Independent Adjudication Committee.

- Creating a market rather than a prize solves many of the challenges in designing incentives for R&D.
- The commitment is designed not only to reward the first producer to bring a product to market but also to create incentives for continuing R&D to create second-generation products that improve on the original.
- Within this broad framework are a number of detailed design choices and variants that should be considered. This will require further discussion among the stakeholders as the details of the commitment are decided.

4

Legal issues: the contract structure

The advance market commitment would derive its credibility—and thus its ability to influence investment behavior—from the legal enforceability of the contracts. This is essential to provide enough assurances to developers to induce them to undertake the large investment for developing a new product.

The challenge is to design contracts sufficiently fixed to ensure that the donors cannot renege on their commitment when a vaccine is developed, but still flexible enough to accommodate contingencies not foreseen when the rules were established.

Working with experienced contract lawyers specializing in the pharmaceutical industry we have drawn up draft term sheets to illustrate the proposed contract (appendixes F and G). These are based on standard contract law, and the component parts of the proposed legal structure are common in law and business.

Some elements of the contract design and incentive structure will depend on the particular product for which the advance market commitment is implemented. But some core elements should be common to advance market commitments, whether for late-stage or early-stage products.

Sponsors, developers and suppliers

Four parties are fundamental to the design—and eventual success—of the advance market commitment. The first is the sponsor—the entity that accepts the contractual obligations associated with funding the market demand. This may be one or more nongovernmental or government grant-making organizations, and must be a legal entity. The second is a developer—one or more pharmaceutical or biotech companies interested in pursuing the contract offered by the sponsor. The third is a designated supplier—that is, one or more developers who actually end up signing the agreement to supply the targeted product. For some products, particularly late-stage products, a single developer may also be the designated supplier. The fourth are the governments of developing countries that would benefit from the vaccines.

Legally binding bilateral contracts

A bilateral contract is one signed by two parties: it becomes binding on the parties as soon as they exchange adequate consideration, which may be in the form of mutual promises, and it allows either party to pursue standard contract remedies, such as money dam-ages and specific performance, if the other party fails to satisfy its contractual commitments. The bilateral structure, as distinct from a unilateral offer or a prize, creates enforceable obligations, making the funding commitment of the sponsor more credible.

The advance market commitment involves two types of legally binding agreements:

- First, an open agreement—the Framework Agreement—indicating the availability of a reward for any firms producing a product meeting pre-specified conditions. In this case, the reward is the right to sign the second contract (appendix F), which will be attached to, and incorporated into, the Framework Agreement. Firms interested in pursuing the R&D of a qualifying product, regardless of whether they are presently doing so, may sign on to this agreement, creating a binding obligation on the part of the sponsor to enter into the Guarantee Agreement with any firm that delivers a qualifying product.
- Second, a bilateral procurement agreement or Guarantee Agreement (appendix G).

The contractual commitments of the sponsor are clear from the outset to provide the promised reward: making co-payments at the guaranteed price, upon satisfaction of the eligibility criteria. Requirements on the developers under the Framework Agreement are minimal. If they succeed in developing a qualifying product, they are entitled to sign the Guarantee Agreement. Under this agreement, in return for being able to sell a number of doses of vaccine at the guaranteed price, the developer guarantees to supply the vaccine to eligible countries at a sustainable low price.

For early-stage products, it is important to have an open agreement at the outset—the Framework Agreement—so that many firms can compete to develop a product.

But for late-stage products, where the market landscape (such as first-generation suppliers and the time lag to second-generation candidates) and product profile are already known with some certainty, it is possible to proceed directly to the Guarantee Agreement, in which the sponsors underwrite a price guarantee.

The Framework Agreement

The Framework Agreement establishes the rules for the competition among potential vaccine developers. Issued by the sponsors, it must be signed by the companies to become binding. At this stage there are only minimal obligations on the part of the signing companies. The Framework Agreement creates the mechanism for the company to enforce the sponsors' commitment to move to a Guarantee Agreement for qualifying products.

The Framework Agreement also sets forth eligibility requirements for the vaccine (§8), creating an Independent Adjudication Committee (IAC) to adjudicate whether the requirements have been met by any candidate vaccine (§13–18) and establishing the rules for legal recourse (§27–29). Finally, the Framework Agreement specifies the incentive mechanism: that a developer of a vaccine meeting the technical specifications and usability requirements is entitled to enter the Guarantee Agreement with the sponsor (§5) (appendix F).

The Guarantee Agreement

The Guarantee Agreement is a bilateral contract between the sponsor and any winners from the open stage (or designated suppliers). The sponsor must irrevocably guarantee that the designated supplier receives the pre-specified reward (price guarantee) for any qualified sales, subject to some also pre-specified cap on the sponsor's total commitment (§3). Qualified sales would be restricted to those that meet criteria established in the original commitment (for example, that the vaccine will be used in a Vaccine Fund–eligible country) (§6).

Guarantee Agreements could be signed with one designated supplier or with multiple suppliers, depending on the rules set out in the Framework Agreement, which would in turn depend on the objectives of the sponsors (§1). The Guarantee Agreement must also specify contract terms related to intellectual property rights, where relevant (§9) (appendix G).

The Independent Adjudication Committee

The IAC is an impartial oversight body at the heart of the credibility of the advance market commitment. The IAC will:

- Decide if a product has met the eligibility criteria. It will have the authority to waive or modify technical specifications and usability requirements as appropriate, but only to make modifications that can lower the bar to accept vaccines that do not meet the specifications in full. The IAC will not have discretion to raise the bar once the framework offer has been made, except in the limited case of a *force majeure* event, and then only with a super-majority vote, which is subject to judicial review (§22).

- Designate approved regulatory bodies (or more likely, designate an approval mechanism—such as the WHO prequalification process) (§5).
- Be the main point of contact with developers throughout the competition.

Once a qualifying vaccine has been identified, the IAC will monitor sales, use and performance of approved vaccines and designate new vaccines as approved under the terms of the Framework Agreement (§8).

Importantly, the IAC's operational budget—to be provided by the sponsors—must be independent so that the sponsors are unable to influence the decisions of the committee after establishing the rules of the game (§18). Similarly, there will be straightforward rules allowing the IAC to recruit new members in the case of retirement or death (§13).

The composition of the IAC is critical to the success of advance market commitment. It should consist of a combination of ex-industry, global health experts, vaccine scientists and legal specialists.

In our consultations with industry, firms emphasized the need for a credible adjudication body and expressed concern about the potential for abuse. The rules must be clearly determined in advance, including dispute resolution. There was strong opinion in favor of having current or recent industry experience represented on the committee.

Dispute resolution

It is impossible to foresee everything that may occur during the life of the advance market commitment. A number of scenarios can be imagined in advance and addressed in the contracts, but the most useful approach to the many unknown scenarios is to establish a clear and credible process for making decisions as events unfold.

While most decisions will be made by the IAC, a decision to invoke the *force majeure* clause should be subject to legal recourse through the courts if necessary (§16).

Exit provisions

It may be sensible to include sunset provisions in the contract to allow sponsors to exit after a certain length of time. For example, if 30 years pass and no substantial progress has been made on the product of interest, a vaccine commitment may not be the most useful approach, and the policy would be worth re-evaluating. So, a sunset clause might be included to specify that, at any time after 20 years had passed, sponsors could give notice that they would let the commitment lapse after 10 years, if no vaccine had been developed by then (§25).

Another type of exit provision—a *force majeure* clause—could allow the obligations to end if the disease environment changed enough to obviate or radically reduce the need for the vaccine. Such changes could occur, for example, if other technologies were developed to control the disease, such as vastly better insecticides against the mosquitoes that transmit malaria. To deal with such contingencies, a vaccine commitment might specify that the sponsor's obligation would end if the independent adjudication committee determined that the burden of disease had fallen by more than 50% or 75% (§22).

To avoid the danger that a *force majeure* clause might be used by a sponsor to renege on the commitment, it would be important to:

- Establish clear standards in the Framework Agreement for invoking the *force majeure* provision.
- Vest the authority to invoke this clause with the IAC, which would be chosen for its credibility, rather than the sponsor, which might have a financial interest in the decision.
- Require a super-majority of the IAC—perhaps a three-quarters vote—to invoke such a clause.
- Make any decision to invoke the clause subject to legal challenge.

Eligibility requirements

Eligibility requirements would define the desired product and other elements required of the developer of the desired product to qualify as a designated supplier. Defining appropriate eligibility requirements is critical to the success of the commitment.

The eligibility requirements would be set by the sponsors in advance, after discussion with key stakeholders (see appendix F). The requirements might include:

- Technical requirements on the product: indication, target population, minimum efficacy requirements, duration of protection, interference.
- Usability requirements on the product: dosage, route of immunization, presentation, storage, safety requirements.
- Specifications of regulatory approval and quality control.

Because these would become the targets of research and product development once established, the framework agreement must not allow sponsors to make the requirements more demanding after it is established. Since products may be useful without perfectly matching all eligibility criteria, the adjudication committee might be given authority to relax the requirements to accept products that nearly meet the pre-established requirement (§5).

In addition, sponsors may establish eligibility requirements on "qualified sales" of a product—for example, that products be sold to a UN agency, developing country or other approved buyer, or that products must be used in a Vaccine Fund or other eligible country. These too must be clearly established from the outset—and must not be subsequently changed to become more onerous.

In our consultations with industry, we found that firms were in favor of setting the bar on product specifications high enough that the sponsor could have reasonable assurance that the product would serve public health needs and be accepted by the relevant developing-country governments. There was also a consensus that there should be a procedure to make the specifications less onerous in case a useful product were developed that did not completely meet all specifications. Industry representatives indicated that they should have the opportunity to review and provide input on product specifications before those specifications were set.

Some firms wanted the opportunity to engage in a dialogue with the adjudication committee during the development process to determine whether the committee would be likely to grant waivers from the stated eligibility guidelines and to learn more about how those guidelines would be interpreted. (This is similar to procedures under which firms have the opportunity to consult the U.S. Food and Drug Administration so that they may structure their pivotal clinical trials and prepare drug approval applications so as to meet better the expectations of the regulatory authority that will be responsible for approving their products.)

Some public health experts were concerned that it would be difficult to establish in advance technical requirements that a vaccine would need to meet. Clearly, it is difficult to say in advance exactly what the characteristics of a successful vaccine will be. But there was a consensus that, if the requirements were framed as outputs rather than a specification of inputs, it would be possible—though complicated—to agree to product requirements in advance. For example, while it would not be desirable to specify in advance whether a malaria vaccine should be a "blood stage" vaccine, it would make sense for the specification to include some minimum duration of protection against severe malaria.

Co-payment and the case against quantity guarantee

We concluded that the advance market commitment should guarantee a minimum price for the vaccine but should not guarantee a minimum quantity that would be bought from each supplier at this price. In this way, the commitment is a market not a prize. There are several reasons why we concluded this was preferable.

The case against a quantity guarantee and for co-payment

First, a quantity guarantee would greatly complicate the drafting of the technical specifications—and perhaps make it impossible. It is possible that a product might meet all the pre-announced eligibility requirements and still be unsuitable for use in poor countries. For example, if a vaccine generated side effects that were medically harmless but culturally unacceptable, there might be an unwillingness to use the vaccine. Attempts to impose its use might even be counterproductive, reducing the acceptability of vaccination in general. It is impossible to anticipate all the possible contingencies in which the purchase of a seemingly effective vaccine would not be warranted, and consequently it is not possible to attempt to write them into the technical specifications. We concluded that the commitment should be to pay for vaccine only if there is demand for the vaccine and if a recipient country is willing to take the steps necessary to ensure that the product is delivered to those who need it. This ensures that sponsors do not find themselves legally obliged to spend $3 billion on a vaccine that nobody wants.

A modest co-payment, either from the country or from a donor, will provide a market test of interest in the vaccine and reduce the risk of waste. As is now the case, a donor could provide the payment through development assistance.

A second benefit of not guaranteeing to buy a particular quantity is that it avoids the problem of deciding what to do if several competing products are successfully introduced. If a superior product becomes available and so qualifies for the price guaranteed under the advance market commitment, the developing countries can choose to use the product most appropriate for their

circumstances because donors are not locked in to paying for a particular quantity from a particular producer.

Our proposed approach of creating a market rather than a prize therefore greatly simplifies the problems that would otherwise occur in trying to draw up a specification that anticipates all eventualities, and in trying to create room for superior products to be developed to enter the market.

Keeping the co-payment low

A disadvantage of the co-payment is that it may add a small amount of uncertainty about whether a product will eventually be purchased, and so may increase the firms' perception of demand risk. This suggests that co-payments should be modest.

Furthermore, requiring a large co-payment might limit access to the product, and by reducing the prospects of adoption it would also reduce incentives for developers.

In principle, the developing country co-payment should be broadly the same amount per course of treatment as the long-term price of the vaccine under the contract. This ensures that developing countries will be asked to pay an affordable and sustainable low price from the outset, which they can be sure will continue when the commitment is exhausted.

The allocation of demand risk

The absence of a quantity guarantee, and the need for co-payments from developing countries, leave some demand risk in the hands of the developers. Given that our objective is to make investment in medicines for neglected diseases more attractive and less risky, we asked ourselves whether the program would be more successful if sponsors took over all the demand risk.

When we discussed this with industry, there was a good understanding of the case for a price guarantee but no quantity guarantee for early-stage products. This allocation of risk resembles the market for medicines in developed countries, in which ability to pay is relatively favorable but quantities are not guaranteed. In this environment firms must bear the risk that customers will not want their product or that they will lose market share to a better product.

The proposed pricing structure—with a high price paid for the first treatments purchased and a low price thereafter—actually transfers a substantial portion of the demand risk from the firms to the sponsors, since the net present value of the revenues to the company is much more stable that it would be under a single price charged over a longer time period. The spreadsheet model demonstrates that, under a more pessimistic scenario in which it takes 15 years for adoption to reach steady-state levels, and adoption reached levels only 10 percentage points below the DPT3 rates, the program would still generate $2.7 billion in revenue in net present value terms for the vaccine developer (in 2004 dollars), and would cost less than $20 per DALY saved.

It is most efficient for risks to be borne by the party that can manage them best. It is desirable for industry to bear some of the demand risk, so that there is an incentive to focus work on producing the most effective and usable product. Under the advance market commitment we have designed, the sponsors would bear the risks associated with unpredictable donor funding and pressure for low pricing, while leaving industry to manage the risks associated with the usefulness of the product.

The guaranteed price

Chapter 5 looks in more detail at the calculation of the appropriate guaranteed price. The goal is to set a price high enough to accelerate R&D in a vaccine for the disease, but at a level at which the purchase of the vaccine, if and when one is developed, is a cost-effective use of aid resources.

To get the full advantage of the commitment, sponsors would need to commit to an overall price well above the pennies-per-dose now paid for existing vaccines in developing countries. The benefit of low prices is that they ensure access to existing vaccines, but they are not sufficient to generate investment in new vaccines or to ensure that new vaccines are rapidly made available in developing countries. Donors increasingly understand that, for vaccines that have only a small market in affluent countries, it will be necessary for firms to recover their R&D costs through higher prices in developing countries than they charge for existing vaccines.

Two-stage pricing

We recommend a two-stage pricing system. In the first stage, a relatively high price (the "guaranteed price") would be guaranteed up to a fixed maximum of treatments purchased. In return for the right to sell at that higher price for the initial treatments sold, the supplier would be contractually committed to supplying further treatments at a lower price set at a level close to the cost of production (the "base price").

Why have two-stage pricing?

Two-stage pricing is attractive to developing countries and sponsors because it would ensure long-term sustainability of the vaccine program. This ensures that sponsors are not undertaking a long-term commitment to purchase vaccines indefinitely, but rather are making a finite commitment that pays for the risk-adjusted costs of R&D and gearing up production, albeit in a different form. Thereafter, pricing is close to marginal cost, which ensures an efficient level of use.

This price structure would also create a strong incentive for firms to accelerate development, because there would be a more substantial reward for the first developer (who could capture the bulk of the high-price market), while the prospect of capturing part of the high-price market would preserve an incentive for the development of improved vaccines later.

A two-stage pricing structure is also attractive to the vaccine developers, because the front-loading of payments would enable them to recover their investment more quickly and with greater certainty than if they charged a single lower price for more doses over a longer time. We found in our discussions with industry that the proposed two-stage price was both understood and welcome.

How would two-stage pricing be implemented in practice?

In return for receiving the guaranteed price for the initial doses, and so recovering their investment, the designated suppliers will be contractually required to supply subsequent doses to eligible countries at the base price, until generics manufacturers take up production, if reasonable notice of demand is given. If a company is not able or chooses not to fulfill that obligation, it faces financial penalties under the contract. Alternatively, it would be required to license the technology for use for developing-country markets or to have the technology placed in the public domain to allow generics producers to meet demand instead. Once the guaranteed price commitment is satisfied, the donors are under no obligation to buy any doses at the base price, but the supplier is under an obligation to meet demand at that price.

The guaranteed (higher) price will be set in advance in the Framework Agreement, at the outset of the commitment. The Framework Agreement will specify how it is to be adjusted for inflation. The price will vary according to the disease.

The base (lower) price can either be set in advance as a dollar amount per treatment or determined by an agreed formula related to the cost of production. There are advantages and disadvantages to each approach. It would be possible to devise more complex hybrid options—for example, in which the sponsors and the producers share the benefits of reducing the cost of production through a formula.

Setting the long-term base price is a critical component of the advance market commitment. Although this is not uncomplicated, we believe that it will be possible to agree an appropriate price, or formula, that is affordable for developing countries while covering the cost of production.

Allowing second entrants but avoiding "me too" copies

The advance market commitment is intended to create a market, not simply to reward the first supplier. We recommend that second and subsequent vaccine suppliers be allowed to compete for the market as designated suppliers, if their products are deemed (by the Independent Adjudication Committee) to be superior, at least in some relevant respect, to existing qualifying products.

Allowing second qualifiers

The ease with which second and subsequent products can qualify needs to balance, on the one hand, the need to avoid creating incentives that lead to wasteful duplication of research that does not lead to improvements, and, on the other hand, the need to ensure that there is scope for incremental improvements as the technology improves. Our proposal—that qualifying vaccines be allowed to enter the market if they can demonstrate that they are superior—is intended to balance these considerations.

It is possible that several different products will be licensed at about the same time. In this case it would be sensible to allow them to share the market at the outset. To achieve this, the contract could allow a window—say one year—within which second qualifying products would be eligible for the guarantee without having to demonstrate superiority.

Sharing the guaranteed market among more than one supplier

The guaranteed price is limited to a fixed number of treatments, even if there is more than one qualifying product. In other words, if there were more than one designated supplier and countries split their demand across the suppliers, no single firm would sell the full designated number of treatments at the guaranteed price.

Once the designated number of treatments has been bought, under the contract suppliers would be required to provide vaccines at a lower price. But at that stage, no supplier would have received the full revenue of the advance market commitment.

We therefore propose that, if a designated supplier has not yet received a pre-determined minimum revenue (which would be less than the total advance market commitment), it be allowed to charge a fixed mark-up over the agreed base price, until its total revenues reach that minimum revenue.

Should we improve the terms over time?

Some industry representatives suggested that sponsors could establish an initial contract but then improve the offer depending on market response. One suggestion was that sponsors could be encouraged to add to the market reward as a successful candidate emerges. Firms with a promising candidate would then be motivated to invest in more expensive trials to reach the growing market. Others suggested that prices or other contract terms be made more attractive to industry over time if the initial terms do not generate the expected response.

This approach has many of the attributes of an auction, which could identify low-cost producers. If the price did not rise too quickly, this would not lead to strategic delay. The Working Group felt that this approach did not have to be included in the initial contract and that it would be open to the sponsors to add it later.

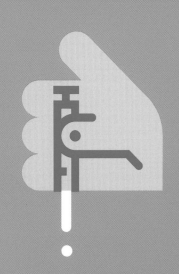

5
$3 billion
per disease

Chapter at a glance

- Our aim is to set a market size large enough to attract serious commercial investment from several pharmaceutical companies that see technological opportunites, while ensuring that the cost of the vaccines purchased is less than the social value and better value for money than alternative uses for the funds.

- A market of $3.1 billion is comparable to the value of lifetime sales of an average pharmaceutical product. Given that expected sales for existing products were sufficient to attract commercial investment from pharmaceutical firms, we recommend commitments worth about $3 billion per disease for early stage products such as malaria.

- Our recommendation is not based on any estimated cost of vaccine R&D. It is based on the realized sales revenues of existing commercial products.

- As an example, taking account of (modest) expected revenues from other markets, a price of $15 per malaria treatment, for 200 million treatments, would provide this revenue and would be exceptionally good value for money in terms of health cost-effectiveness.

- Larger commitments would likely further accelerate development of vaccines; even with higher costs, vaccines would still be a bargain in development spending.

Determining the size of the market needed

Goals

In setting the parameters of the advance market commitment, the sponsors should aim to:

- Set the guaranteed market revenue high enough to accelerate R&D in the selected vaccine.
- Set the size of the commitment below the social value of the vaccine, so that the sponsors do not commit themselves to paying more for the vaccine than it is worth to society. Specifically, the commitment should be low enough that spending on the vaccine is cost-effective compared with alternative development interventions.

It turns out that there is a large window between these lower and upper bounds for setting a commitment. In other words, a wide range of guaranteed prices and maximum quantities would give firms a good return on investment in R&D and still represent an excellent bargain for sponsors seeking to maximize the effectiveness of their spending.

We do not believe that the optimal market commitment is the minimum level needed to lead to a vaccine eventually being developed, even if we thought there were some way to estimate this. If a larger market commitment is likely to lead to a vaccine being developed more quickly, with greater certainty or with more competition, accelerating the development of a vaccine by paying more for it would likely be a very good investment. The optimal market size, therefore, is likely to be somewhat above the minimum R&D cost needed to develop the vaccine.

What market size is needed to accelerate vaccine development?

The larger the expected value of the potential market, the more firms will enter the field, the more research leads each firm will pursue and the faster a product is likely to be developed. In light of the enormous health burden imposed by diseases such as malaria, it is important to provide sufficient incentives for multiple researchers to enter the field and to induce major pharmaceutical firms to pursue many avenues of research simultaneously so that vaccines can be developed quickly.

In other words, the more sponsors are willing to commit to pay, the greater will be the likely number of firms, the larger those firms' investments and the faster the development of a vaccine. Even though we cannot reliably predict how much faster a vaccine would be developed as a result of increased investments, both evidence and theory tell us that total commercial investments would be expected to rise with the increase in expected market size.[1]

We decided to calibrate the appropriate value for each advance market commitment by looking at the net present value of sales revenues of existing commercial products, the expected sales of which clearly motivated biotech and pharmaceutical companies to invest in the past.

The most recent comprehensive data on sales revenues for pharmaceutical products look at 118 new medicines introduced in the United States between 1990 and 1994.[2] Our analysis uses this sales revenue data and finds that the average net present value of lifetime sales revenue for products in that sample is $3.1 billion (in 2004 dollars).[3]

Vaccine suppliers would earn some revenues from sources other than sales under the purchase commitment. For a malaria vaccine effective against the form of malaria endemic to Africa there would be sales to travelers and the military, and to the private sector in poor countries. We estimate that the net present value of purchases in these markets would be about $850 million, so an advance market commitment would need to create a market of approximately $2.3 billion in expected revenue to create total expected revenues of $3.1 billion.[4]

Note that this is not an estimate of the cost of R&D for a new vaccine. It is simply an approximate measure of the realized sales revenues of the average of a sample of products whose expected sales were sufficient to spur R&D investments from pharmaceutical companies in the past.

We therefore conclude that an advance market commitment offering total market revenues of about $3.1 billion (as a net present value) could be expected to stimulate pharmaceutical companies to invest in R&D on a commercial basis.

What price would guarantee a return of $3 billion?

For a malaria vaccine, under fairly pessimistic assumptions on uptake rates, this might correspond to a commitment to pay $15 (in today's prices) for each of the first 200 million people immunized under the program.

Other combinations of price and quantity are possible. A lower price, with a correspondingly higher maximum quantity to which the guarantee applies, would create a smaller degree of front-loading of the return. This might be preferable to the extent that the first product to market is likely to be imperfect, and it is important to create incentives for improved products.

Some firms that we spoke to suggested a flexible pricing mechanism (such as cost plus some mark-up) instead of trying to set a price in advance. The rationale for this is that it is difficult to predict which technologies will succeed and thus to anticipate the cost of production. Firms could be sheltered from some of this risk through cost-plus pricing, albeit with a corresponding increase in the risk to sponsors. But this approach would reduce incentives to develop products that could be produced cheaply or to develop inexpensive manufacturing processes—and it might add uncertainty to the commitment. Moreover, if a product were too expensive, it would not be a cost-effective use of a sponsor's funds to purchase it. For simplicity, the term sheets include a simple cost-plus formula, subject to a cap.

What price is worth paying for vaccines?

Developing countries—and donors on their behalf—currently pay less than $0.50 a dose for most vaccines. This has the advantage of reducing the cost to highly stretched health budgets. But as set out in chapter 1, it means that the introduction of new vaccines to poor countries is significantly delayed and that there is insufficient incentive to develop new vaccines for diseases in developing countries.

Some of the most significant benefits of an advance market commitment would come from enhancing the size and predictability of the market, by committing to pay a price for new medicines that meets the cost of innovation. In fact, a guaranteed price considerably higher than pennies-per-dose would still be highly cost-effective relative to other health, and other development, policies.

We used malaria as an example to illustrate the orders of magnitude involved. Consider a commitment to purchase a malaria vaccine at a price of $15 (in today's prices) per person immunized for the first 200 million people immunized. This commitment, together with estimated revenues from other markets, provides an expected return to developers of approximately $3.1 billion, comparable to average revenue for commercial products as discussed

above. In return for this revenue, the developers guarantee to sell subsequent treatments at $1 each.

The cost-effectiveness of such a commitment would depend on a number of assumptions. These assumptions were employed for the example developed by the Working Group, and should be refined with additional analyses and consultations. To get an idea of the magnitudes, assume that:

- The contract covers all countries with a GNP of less than $1,000 a year with sufficient disease prevalence to make vaccination worthwhile (in terms of being cost effective at less than $100 per DALY saved; see box 3.1).
- Countries adopt the vaccine over seven years and eventually attain a steady-state immunization level five percentage points above that of the basic childhood immunization program.
- The vaccine requires three doses but could be delivered with the childhood immunization package at an incremental delivery cost of $0.75.
- The vaccine is 60% effective, protects against infection for five years and does not lead to a rebound effect by weakening limited natural immunity.

Given these assumptions and data on population, fertility and disease prevalence, the cost—including incremental delivery costs—per DALY saved would be about $15 (discounted in 2004 dollars), making vaccine purchases under the program one of the world's most cost-effective health interventions.[5]

The value-for-money from such a program is robust to changes in assumptions about efficacy, uptake rates or the price offered. Furthermore, this is a highly conservative estimate of the program's cost-effectiveness. The calculation does not include epidemiological benefits—vaccinating a significant fraction of the population may slow the spread of a disease, and thus benefits may spill over to the unvaccinated. It does not include savings to developing-country health systems from lower rates of illness and morbidity. It does not include health benefits to people in middle- and high-income countries or benefits to adults in low-income countries who purchase a vaccine privately. It assumes that the vaccine would be given randomly throughout a country and thus does not include the efficiency benefits of targeting vaccine delivery within countries to areas that have the most severe disease problems. Finally, it does not include any benefits of increasing vaccination rates for other diseases that might arise if parents know they can vaccinate their children against malaria by bringing them to a clinic.

These estimates demonstrate that, once a vaccine is developed, purchasing it at a price well above current prices paid for vaccines in developing countries would still be one of the most cost-effective health interventions, more cost-effective than a wide range of other development expenditures.

Is the commitment the right size?

If an increase in the size of the commitment would accelerate development of a vaccine, is it worth making a commitment to a higher price or paying for a larger number of doses? For example, paying $17 per person for the first 200 million people immunized rather than $15 per person would increase the overall market size to $3.6 billion, comparable with the revenues for the average drug in the 70th to 80th percentile, at a cost of $16 per DALY saved. Or paying $25 per person immunized for the first 250 million people immunized would increase the overall market size to $5.7 billion, comparable with the average drug in the 80th to 90th percentile of drug revenues, at a cost of about $23 per DALY saved. Either of these commitment sizes would create attractive markets for developers and still be cost-effective from a public health perspective.

These calculations demonstrate that once a vaccine is developed, purchasing a vaccine at the pre-specified price would be very cost-effective. A more complex issue is the value of a commitment in accelerating the development and distribution of a vaccine, which requires assumptions about what would happen in the absence of a commitment. We estimate that if a vaccine purchase commitment advanced vaccine development by 10 years and accelerated access in poor countries by 10 years, it would cost only about $23 per additional DALY saved. Even in the extreme case in which a price commitment accelerated vaccine development by only one year and adoption in poor countries by only two years, the program would cost about $80–90 per additional DALY saved—still less than the $100 per DALY cost-effectiveness threshold for the poorest countries.

Hence under a large range of assumptions and contract structures, a vaccine commitment could be priced at a level likely sufficient to stimulate substantial private R&D, yet still be cost-effective from a public health and donor perspective.

A commitment of $15–25 for each of the first 200–250 million people immunized would be a bargain in terms of public health cost-effectiveness. Within this range larger commitments would be expected to lead to more firms to enter the search for a vaccine and shorten the expected time to development and distribution.

Cost-effectiveness of an advance market commitment for HIV and tuberculosis vaccines

A spreadsheet model (available for download from the Center for Global Development website at www.cgdev.org/vaccine) allows users to analyze a large number of different scenarios and estimate the costs and benefits of commitments for malaria, tuberculosis and HIV vaccines under a variety of assumptions, such as about delivery costs, uptake, disease burden and eligibility.[6] Appendix E gives a short overview of the spreadsheet.

We present here estimates produced by this spreadsheet model under a set of conservative benchmark assumptions. Although we have used the example of malaria throughout this report, the spreadsheet estimates similar degrees of cost-effectiveness for commitments to purchase vaccines for tuberculosis or HIV (table 5.1). Note that additional analytic work would be required to refine the estimates.

Malaria has a particularly low cost per DALY because the burden of disease is highly geographically concentrated in Africa and hence it would be possible to economize on delivery costs by targeting the vaccine. However, given that the burden of disease from tuberculosis and HIV is estimated to exceed that of malaria,

Table 5.1
Cost-effectiveness of an advance market commitment of $3.1 billion

Disease	Estimated cost per DALY would be less than . . .
Malaria	$15
HIV	$17
Tuberculosis	$30

Source: Spreadsheet model available at www.cgdev.org/vaccine.

the cost per DALY alone should not be the sole determinant of policy priorities.

The International AIDS Vaccine Initiative and the Malaria Vaccine Initiative are both conducting more detailed investigations of the appropriate parameters for an advance market commitment for a vaccine for each of those diseases, with the aim of making recommendations for how the commitment should be tailored to the circumstances of those diseases.

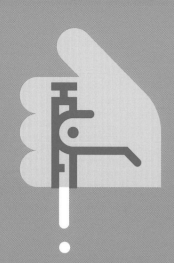

6
Meeting industry requirements

Chapter at a glance

- We have sought to design a mechanism to which industry will respond by increasing R&D on vaccines for diseases occurring mainly in developing countries.
- Industry is attracted to the concept of payment for results; the market mechanism fits their business model well and preserves the role of intellectual property rights and market sales financing commercial investment in pharmaceutical R&D.
- Our consultations revealed a range of priorities for the commitment from different parts of industry.
- An advance market commitment would be of value to developing-country suppliers, which often do not benefit from other incentive arrangements.
- Complementary measures are needed to improve the procurement of existing vaccines, improve demand forecasts and increase funding for existing drugs and vaccines.

A range of industry requirements

The success of the advance market commitment depends on creating effective incentives for potential vaccine developers and suppliers who see a scientific potential to invest. The program is intended to create incentives to accelerate the development of new vaccines, but the details of the design may make a significant difference to the incentives that the contract creates. Critical determinants of success include the size of the reward, the contractual requirements placed on the firm (for example, the eligibility requirements) and the public relations impact of participation.

We have borne in mind that our goal is not to encourage all firms to work on these products. It is to accelerate the development of a vaccine by providing sufficient incentive for some firms to begin R&D on these problems, and for others to devote extra resources and priority to their existing work.

Initial research often is done by biotech companies. Typically, their work is then either licensed to, or bought by, larger pharmaceutical companies for the later stages of development, marketing and manufacturing. An important ingredient in the proposal is that it should generate a response from biotechs and other early-stage researchers—for example, by creating a sufficient market for the vaccine to give them confidence that pharmaceutical companies will invest in intermediate research outputs. Biotech companies and venture capitalists would be more willing to invest because they would be more confident that they would attract interest from pharmaceutical companies for the products they develop. There is considerable evidence that firms do, in fact, respond to market signals by adjusting their R&D to reflect the size of the potential market.[1]

The only way to know for sure how firms would react is to implement a commitment and observe what happens. In the meantime, it is possible to obtain information through structured consultations with informed individuals, particularly those who are currently facing difficult choices about where to invest in R&D to yield the best outcome for shareholders. We consulted representatives of three industry groups—biotechnology firms of various sizes and orientations, multinational vaccine manufacturers and emerging market suppliers (box 6.1). We sought feedback on the overall concept and tried to identify specific ways in which the advance contract concept could be structured to most likely generate a change in investment behavior. The results of these

discussions, summarized here, were invaluable for developing our recommendations. Our aim has been to design a commitment that creates the right commercial incentives to encourage industry to invest, while ensuring value for money for sponsors.

The industry is diverse

Firms had various reactions to the idea of an advance commitment, depending on their risk tolerance, product pipeline, scientific background and business model. There was a greater degree of consistency within industry categories, but even within these categories each firm indicated a unique character and strategic agenda. For example, pharmaceutical companies with vaccines coming to market soon were more interested in commitments for late-stage products than were biotechs engaged in research on early-stage products.

Many firms expressed a view that an advance market commitment, if structured in the right way, would be exactly what they needed to make the case for keeping global health products in the development pathway. Others felt there was little commercial motivation that could stimulate a dramatic change in their research pipelines.

Although some have interpreted advance market commitments to be targeted at multinational firms, emerging suppliers from developing countries would also have the potential to benefit. Unlike some incentives that would benefit primarily large and profitable pharmaceutical companies (U.S. tax credits, transferable patents), all firms would be in a position to compete for the market offered by this commitment. Major vaccine firms in Brazil,

---

Box 6.1
Industry consultations

- Biotechs: Ardana, Avant, Human Genome Sciences, Maxygen, Mojave Therapeutics, Nectar Therapeutics, Targeted Genetics, Vertex.
- Multinational vaccine manufacturers: Aventis-Pasteur, Chiron, GSK Biologicals, Merck Vaccine Division, Wyeth.
- Emerging supplier: Serum Institute of India.

In addition, the Working Group spoke with several former senior industry executives.

India, Indonesia and elsewhere that have demonstrated the capacity to achieve tremendous scale efficiencies of production could participate through joint ventures or other types of partnerships with firms that have a strong tradition of innovation.

Key industry requirements

Some themes emerged from the consultations.

- A commitment is likely to have more impact on some firms than others. For products at an early stage, for example, an advance market commitment may initially motivate biotech companies and the venture capitalists that provide their funding, while some larger multinational pharmaceutical firms may get involved only after further advances in the science, perhaps led by biotech firms.

- For many firms the establishment of a significant financial reward for the successful developer would be important in within-firm analysis and in negotiations about which products to move ahead with and at what pace. These firms cited in particular the moments in the development pathway when relatively costly decisions are taken to test products in humans.

- Some respondents indicated that an advance market commitment would address industry concerns about the appropriation of intellectual property and the downward pressure on prices that occurs when an essential medicine is developed but is seen as unaffordable to the developing world.

- Commercial decisions to develop a particular candidate are based on market prospects but also—critically—on science. Access to a promising scientific pathway will be the primary determinant of some firms' investment decisions in early research. There was a wide range of opinions about the challenges of developing a malaria vaccine, for example, and some firms reported that they are unwilling to invest given the current state of science. The public sector will need to keep investing in basic research and lead development to advance the science.

- Firms do not evaluate incentives independently but look at the comprehensive picture of risks and rewards they will face through the development process.

- An advance market commitment, or indeed any similar mechanism focused on creating incentives for commercial investment, would need to be implemented in coordination with other interventions—push funding, demand creation and capacity-building for distribution and delivery.

- Weaknesses in the current system of procurement and delivery of vaccines for the developing world are a major deterrent to investment. Most firms supplying developing-country markets through public procurement are frustrated with inefficiencies in the current system—short-term purchase agreements, the lack of enforceable contracts, unreliable demand forecasts and underuse of existing vaccines. The public sector can improve its credibility by increasing use of existing products and by improving demand forecasts.

- The credibility of the commitment is closely related to the credibility of the sponsor. Citing real-world examples, firms were not convinced of the public sector's ability to live up to its funding promises that are not legally binding. Firms indicated that the inclusion of a private foundation as sponsors would add enormously to the credibility of the proposal. It was therefore clear from the consultations that it would be essential for an advance market commitment to be legally binding on the sponsors, and that nonbinding statements of intent would not elicit the same response.

- Given the novelty of the advance market commitment for the public sector, industry will be most persuaded by successful execution. Firms expressed uniform enthusiasm for implementing long-term contracts for late-stage (and existing) products. In addition to being directly beneficial by increasing affordable access to those vaccines, this would build up the credibility of similar commitments for early-stage products.

We have looked carefully at each of these industry considerations and sought to ensure that our advance market proposal takes these concerns into account. Firms also gave specific feedback on the proposed structure of advance contracts, particularly the Framework Agreement and Guarantee Agreement. These points have been taken into account in the advance market proposal set out in chapters 3 and 4 and are reflected in the discussion in those chapters.

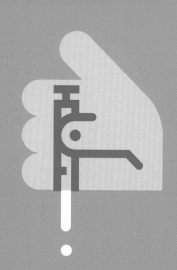

7
How sponsors can do it

Chapter at a glance

- Government sponsors can make legally binding commitments—and do so all the time. Private sponsors can too, and their involvement would add to the credibility of the commitment.
- The commitment can be handled within existing government budget processes.
- Under normal accounting rules for the sponsors included in the analysis, there is no cost to sponsors until and unless a vaccine is developed.
- There is no short-term budgetary tradeoff with existing funding of R&D.
- Existing procurement and regulatory arrangements can be used.

- An advance market commitment will require the sponsors to enter into an agreement, enforceable by law, to make multiyear payments of uncertain size and duration (though with a known upper limit) to an unknown recipient at some unknown time in the future. Can sponsors, as matter of practical fact, make a commitment of this sort? We looked at whether there are any institutional or legal obstacles to making commitments and how such commitments would be treated in the budget process. We found that there are no obstacles to sponsors making this commitment.

Possible government sponsors

The United States

We start with the United States because its budgetary process is more complicated than that of other possible sponsors.

The starting point is that the U.S. government enters long-term contracts as a matter of course. An administration is able to enter legal agreements that bind its successors. The government has budgeting mechanisms to authorize and deliver multi-year funding streams in the future. These obligations are legally binding and credible in markets even in the face of a degree of uncertainty about the appropriations process. Indeed, U.S. law specifically waives U.S. sovereign immunity for contracts executed by the United States in its proprietary capacity.

An example of a legally binding government commitment is the sale of government bonds, contracts that oblige the government to pay money to bondholders in the future. The U.S. government faces no legal difficulty making such commitments, even though they bind successor administrations.

To enter a contractual commitment to buy vaccines in the future, the administration needs specific authority from Congress. Once that legal authority exists, the mechanics of signing a legally binding commitment are uncomplicated.

A U.S. government commitment to purchase vaccines, even one that is legally binding, would not score as government expenditure, or contribute to the government deficit, until the vaccine is produced and purchased. Until then, the commitment remains a long-term liability and (depending on the perceived probability of the vaccine being developed) would be included in long-term projections of outlays.

But for the administration to sign the contract, it would need approval from Congress, and the measure granting this approval would score against the congressional appropriations ceiling within which budgets are set.

If other budget lines had to be reduced to accommodate a commitment within a fixed appropriations ceiling, the commitment would require changes elsewhere in the budget: current programs, delivering certain and immediate benefits, would have to be reduced to make way for the uncertain future benefits of the advance markets commitment. Such an approach would be unlikely to command political support.

But with sufficient political will, this can be overcome within the U.S. budget framework. One practical approach is for the authorizing legislation to be made outside the appropriations process, for example, by the Energy and Commerce Committee. In the best case, the congressional budget plan would explicitly accommodate the budget authority needed for the program. This might be reasonably straightforward to agree, because the budget authority needed for that committee would not compete with the authority needed for the Appropriations Committee, and the expenditure authorized would have no impact on outlay projections (over the time horizon of the projections) or on the deficit.

Even if Congress did not include the advance market commitment in the budget, the Energy and Commerce Committee could seek approval for the legislation later in the year. By bringing the legislation outside the Appropriations Committee, the focus of attention would be on the impact on the outlay projections (none), not on the budget authority needed. And congressional leadership might well agree to waive the budget ceilings in this instance.

There are other possible approaches to securing budget authority for the necessary legislation without competing with other more immediate spending priorities. If the Appropriations Committee felt that, for reasons of precedent, it would be preferable for the authority to be provided by an appropriations bill, Congress could budget for a one-off, ring-fenced bulge in the appropriations ceiling to accommodate the commitment. Given that the commitment would have no impact on outlay or deficit projections, a one-off change to the appropriations ceiling to accommodate the commitment would be relatively easy to defend.

We conclude that the treatment in the U.S. budget system is not straightforward, and approval will depend on there being sufficient political support for the proposal. But we also believe that this is a policy with broad bipartisan appeal, and that with some political leadership, it could secure the commitment necessary to navigate the budget process.

We are clear, however, that if there is political support for the idea, there is no technical obstacle that would prevent the U.S. government from making a long-term advance market commitment.

The United Kingdom

The U.K. government, through the Department for International Development (DFID), could commit to an advance market within its existing budget mechanisms.

While there is no precedent in DFID for making legally binding commitments to procure products that do not yet exist, it has implemented innovative financing approaches that have similar characteristics. Examples include trust funds, endowments and provisions for guarantees, as well as statements of intent to provide long-term funding support for country programs. DFID has issued guarantees to a company operating on a capital aid project to meet the costs of certain disputed claims (£30 million). Other contingent liabilities on the books include the United Kingdom's share of callable capital at the International Bank for Reconstruction and Development (€5.5 billion) and government guarantees to international financial institutions for U.K. loans to dependent territories (£2.4 billion).

The International Development Act of 2002 empowered the Secretary of State to use "non-grant financial instruments including guarantees" in pursuit of the department's objectives. No further specific legislative authority is required for DFID to enter a commitment of the kind envisaged for an advance market.

An advance market commitment in the U.K. budget

The scoring of expenditure in the U.K. budget is intended to closely follow private sector accounting rules. Under U.K. accounting rules, as set out in FRS 12,[1] the advance market commitment would be deemed to be an executory contract (that is, a contract in which both parties have not yet fully performed their obligations). Under FRS 12, obligations under contracts to make or take future supplies of goods and services do not normally need to be included on the balance sheet, and so do not give rise to contingent liabilities or require the body to take a provision.

The main exception is an "onerous contract," in which the unavoidable costs of meeting the obligations under it exceed the economic benefits expected to be received from it. As seen in chapter 5, the economic benefits of the advance market commitment exceed the cost, so the commitment is not onerous and would not require DFID to include a contingent liability or provision in the balance sheet.

Because an advance market commitment would not have to be included on the department's balance sheet, there would be no need to make budgetary provision at the time the commitment was made, and there would be no short-term cost for DFID. If and when a vaccine was available and spending actually occurred, DFID would be required to meet the costs from within its budget granted by parliament. For a given expenditure limit, this would require lower spending elsewhere. (This is discussed in the box on budgetary tradeoffs later in this chapter.)

The U.K. government has chosen to base its overall fiscal framework, including targets for spending and the deficit, on national accounts measures. The expenditure would not be recorded in the U.K. national accounts until the government was actually buying vaccines.

Other governments

We have not looked in detail at the arrangements for other governments, but we believe that the main donor countries could, if they chose, make an advance market commitment consistent with their normal legal and budgetary processes.

The World Bank

The International Development Association (IDA) of the World Bank, which provides subsidized loans and grants, could in principle also be a sponsor of an advance market commitment.[2] But the normal operation of World Bank lending would need to be modified.

Forward commitment

Sponsors would need to make a legally binding commitment, perhaps 10 or more years in advance of the likely spending. But the priorities for IDA loans and grants are usually set only over a five-year time horizon, and the World Bank has been reluctant to earmark specific sums for specific programs.

There does not appear to be any legal impediment to the World Bank's legally binding itself to provide IDA loans or grants to any member state that wants to purchase the vaccine under the advance market commitment. This would, however, be a departure from current practice—and may be thought to set unwelcome precedents for earmarking. However, in principle this would be a commitment different in character from other earmarking proposals, because it is a contract to buy specific goods in the future, and so it may be possible to prevent it from setting a more general precedent.

Loans or grants?

IDA loans, which are at below-market rates, carry an implicit subsidy of roughly 60%.[3] Since the bulk of the expense of purchasing the vaccine represents the cost of research and development, which is a global public good, it is appropriate for these costs to be met from grants rather than the 40% co-payment by developing countries implicit in IDA terms. This could be achieved through IDA if the World Bank were to increase the subsidy on the loans (reduce recipient countries' co-payment) by offsetting part of the vaccine purchase price through grants.

Alternatively, other donors—either private foundations or governments—could make a commitment to "buy down" IDA loans used to purchase vaccine. In other words, they could give the member money to repay the loan—as for Nigeria's polio eradication campaign. One particularly attractive element of this buy-down approach is that governments or private foundations could deposit promissory notes with a World Bank trust fund now but would not need to make payments until appropriate vaccines were developed and IDA loans were extended for purchases. Where national budgeting rules are amenable, the commitment would not count toward government outlays until the funds were drawn.

Additionality

For the commitment to be effective, the World Bank would need to agree in advance that IDA loans and grants for purchasing vaccines under the advance market commitment would be additional to the IDA allocation for the country using them. Otherwise, since countries are restricted in the value of IDA credits they can use in a single year, it is possible that developing countries would be reluctant to purchase vaccines, since this would use up a portion of their IDA allocation, which they might need for other purposes.

At present, all IDA is allocated to country programs. There is no procedure to set aside funds for global public goods. To ensure that IDA funding of purchases under an advance market commitment was genuinely additional, it would be necessary if and when a vaccine is developed to set aside some funds that were not taken from country allocations. Again, while there is no precedent for this, there are no legal obstacles to doing so.

Foundations

Given that the advance market commitment is a straightforward contract, there are no legal or budgetary obstacles that would prevent private foundations from making an advance market commitment.

The budgetary implications for an endowment-based foundation are a bit different from the considerations for a government with indefinite tax revenues. An advance market commitment represents a claim on a portion of the endowment, which means that the money cannot also be spent in another way. But foundations invest the majority of their principal in any case. This principal, invested to earn a return for the foundation, would also serve as the asset underpinning the commitment—in effect, the foundation can put the same funds to work twice in the interests of the poor.

In the short run, before a vaccine is available, and provided that the foundation's total commitment is less than the principal that the foundation plans to invest in any case, this commitment would have no effect on the foundation's revenue or expenditures.

If and when the vaccine is produced, the foundation will, as a result of the commitment, be required to make co-payments toward the vaccine purchase. At this stage, the foundation may choose to divert spending from other priorities (especially where it expects to make savings as a result of the availability of the vaccine—as for the purchase of drugs or investment in R&D), to cut lower priority programs or to increase its total spending.

Some foundations have a policy against using resources to pay for current goods and services and to avoid undertaking open-ended commitments to meet current costs that should be the obligation of governments. The combination of the dual-price structure and co-payments by developing countries in the advance market commitment means that the donors' contributions correspond to the incentives for commercial investment in R&D and the cost of scaling up large-scale production. The marginal cost of production of the vaccine, which foundations may as a matter of policy not wish to fund, is accounted for by the developing countries' co-payments. So although the contract takes the form of the purchase of vaccines, because that is the best way to create the right incentives for effective and well targeted R&D, the contribution of donors is conceptually meeting the cost of the R&D and subsidizing scaling up production. It is therefore quite unlike making an open-ended and unsustainable commitment to meet future vaccine costs.

It would be particularly beneficial to the credibility of the advance market program for private foundations to be sponsors or co-sponsors of the commitment because:

- They have greater continuity of leadership and strategic focus, so they are perceived as less likely to change direction.
- They may be perceived to be less vulnerable to lobbying from special interest groups.
- They have a substantial asset base and no ability to legislate away their obligations, so their commitment is regarded as highly reliable.

The Global Alliance on Vaccines and Immunization and the Vaccine Fund

The mandate of the Global Alliance on Vaccines and Immunization

The Global Alliance for Vaccines and Immunization (GAVI) is an alliance between the private and public sector, with the mission of saving children's lives and protecting people's health through the widespread use of vaccines. GAVI brings together governments in developing and industrialized countries, established and emerging vaccine manufacturers, nongovernmental organizations, research institutes, the United Nations Children's Fund (UNICEF), the World Health Organization, the Bill & Melinda Gates Foundation and the World Bank.

GAVI has a unique role in increasing resources allocated to the purchase and use of vaccines and in improving the way those resources are used. It focuses on areas in which no one partner can work alone effectively and to add value to what partners are already doing. GAVI's added value has been defined in four areas:

- Coordination and consensus-building.
- Funding support to countries, through the Vaccine Fund. Resources are provided to countries to purchase vaccines and other supplies and to support the operational costs of immunization.
- Innovation—examples include the country proposal and review process, performance-based grants for immunization services support, financial sustainability planning, the Data Quality Audit, Vaccine Provision Project and Accelerated Development and Introduction Plans.
- Advocacy and communications—particularly to inform decisionmaking among policymakers and donors on the

value of vaccination for reducing poverty and infant mortality in the developing world.

There is a strong fit between these four areas and the goals of an advance market commitment. Given their mandates, GAVI and the Vaccine Fund are natural partners in an advance market commitment. In particular, GAVI, or an alliance of members under its auspices, might be an appropriate forum for donors to reach a consensus about the approach, and agree on the details of the commitment. Commitments might then be made by donors directly or through guarantees to the Vaccine Fund, which is a member of GAVI.

The Vaccine Fund could become a sponsor of an advance market commitment, if it were underwritten by its donors to do so. Given the role of the Vaccine Fund in buying vaccines, there would be advantages in structuring financial arrangements to enable it to enter into advance market commitments. Depending on budgetary constraints on the part of the donors, this might take the form of direct financing or suitable (legally binding) guarantees from donors—for example, through the International Finance Facility for Immunization (IFFIm) initiative.

The International Finance Facility

The U.K. Treasury has proposed an International Finance Facility (IFF) to accelerate progress toward the Millennium Development Goals by issuing bonds on international markets. If established, the IFF would:

- Create a financing mechanism that would provide up to an additional $50 billion a year in development assistance until 2015.
- Lever additional money from the international capital markets by issuing bonds based on legally binding long-term donor commitments.
- Repay bondholders using future donor payment streams.
- Disburse resources through existing multilateral and bilateral mechanisms.

The IFF proposal has generated interest and support from emerging markets, developing countries, international institutions, faith communities, nongovernmental organizations and businesses.

The International Finance Facility for Immunization initiative

There are discussions among DFID, the U.K. Treasury and GAVI to consider options for piloting the IFF approach through the

Vaccine Fund. A Working Group, including the Bill & Melinda Gates Foundation, GAVI and the Vaccine Fund, is looking at the technical case for this approach.

IFFIm is intended to create a framework in which:

- Donor funding for vaccines over the next 15 years is planned.
- On the strength of these plans, the initiative is able to program spending over a 10-year horizon.
- Funding for vaccines is therefore better planned, more predictable and delivered sooner.

There are several arguments for front-loading spending on vaccines in the way implied by using IFFIm:

- Having a quicker impact on immunization, thus reducing child mortality, reducing the burden of disease and accelerating economic growth.
- Providing incentives for vaccine producers to invest in production facilities and to develop new vaccines through greater market certainty or a short-term price top-up to allow producers to cover development costs earlier.
- Accelerating of new products through R&D and trials for new vaccines.
- Developing health systems with long-term capacity benefits.

In principle, these characteristics would enable the initiative to secure greater value with the same amount of donor funds, compared with the existing situation of allocating funds from one year to the next.

Using IFFIm to implement an advance market commitment

Like the advance market proposal, IFFIm is based on the idea that by increasing certainty about their future behavior, donors can increase the productivity of their spending. The market for vaccines would be more efficient, providing vaccines to more people at a lower cost, if there were greater certainty of demand, which is presently hampered by unpredictable funding. A more reliable market would enable firms to invest more at every stage of the process, from scientific research, through clinical trials, to investment in production capacity. This would result in new vaccines becoming available more quickly and larger volumes being available more cheaply.

Because it will generate committed funding over 10 years, funds from IFFIm could implement an advance market commitment for new vaccines, such as for rotavirus and pneumococcus.

It might not be appropriate, however, for IFFIm to make a long-term legally binding commitment to vaccines not likely to be available over the next 10 years, as this will be outside its lifespan. There is thus a strong case for a group of donors to make a separate legally binding advance market commitment for vaccines for such diseases as malaria, tuberculosis and HIV, in addition to the proposed commitment to purchasing vaccines through IFFIm.

An advance market commitment as a complementary financing mechanism for IFFIm

The IFFIm financial mechanism requires donors to provide pledges to a financial vehicle, which on the strength of those pledges can borrow in financial markets to rephase and commit that spending. But because of constraints on budget processes, financial accounting or limitations on legal powers, some donors may not be able to make a pledge of this kind.

The advance market commitment is a different kind of arrangement, taking the form of a long-term procurement contract. Most governments have ways to make long-term commitments of this kind, and there are budgetary procedures for this. It is therefore possible that some donors that could not contribute directly through the IFFIm financial mechanism would be able to make an advance market commitment for the purchase of vaccines such as rotavirus and pneumococcus. These commitments could then be taken into account in the overall planning of IFFIm. This provides an alternative way for donors to contribute to the overall IFFIm initiative, even if they are not yet able to contribute through the financial mechanism (figure 7.1 and box 7.1).

Would sponsors pay twice?

Some sponsors with significant portfolios of direct funding of R&D may be concerned that they would end up "paying twice" for R&D on new vaccines: first, when they support R&D and basic science and again when they pay for vaccines under the advance market commitment.

This concern can usefully be put in context. First, the United States and other countries routinely support R&D through public sector and philanthropic programs, and accept that products that benefit from that investment will later be purchased at above marginal cost through Medicare and other public insurance programs. Second, the vast majority of the spending under the advance market commitment—such as late-stage clinical trials, commercial development, regulatory approval through licensure and investments in large-scale productive capacity—currently receives very little support through push-funding mechanisms. So while the advance market commitment would stimulate some R&D in basic science and identification of candidates, the bulk of the revenues from an advance market commitment will cover costs that were incurred on activities that are, for the most part, outside the current scope of push funding. Moreover, the size of the advance market commitment can be set to reflect the extent of the contribution that is being made by push-funded R&D.

However, to the extent that there is duplication, in principle it would be possible to structure either push funding or the advance market commitment to prevent double payment. In practice, it would be very difficult to change the advance market payout according to the origins of the original investment, as this would:

- Require the Independent Adjudication Committee to collect information about the costs, funding and institutional

and intellectual heritage of qualifying products that they would not otherwise have or need.

- Introduce a considerable element of discretion into the operation of the advance market commitment—which would lead to a level of uncertainty that could greatly diminish firms' interest in investing.

- Distort the market for products once they are developed: in particular, sponsors might be inclined to encourage purchase of an inferior product just because it would incur a lower payout as a result of having had more push funding in the past; this would create a bias that might undermine the incentive to buy the best available vaccines when they are available.

By contrast, it might be quite straightforward to adapt push funding arrangements for the existence of an advance market commitment. For example, funders of research could explicitly take the existence of an advance market commitment into consideration when negotiating upfront support or milestone payments. This is done now for development of some products, when there

Figure 7.1
Possible relationship between the International Finance Facility for Immunization initiative and advance market commitment

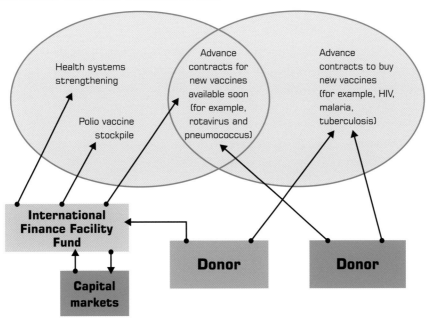

Box 7.1
Is there a budgetary tradeoff?

If sponsors make an advance market commitment, will they need to make corresponding reductions elsewhere, for example in their direct support for R&D?

An advance market commitment would increase commercial investment in R&D, which in turn would increase the productivity of existing and future donor and philanthropic investments in R&D, for at least two reasons. First, there would be a larger and better-resourced scientific community working on the issues, which would benefit everyone engaged in that research. Second, there would be a much higher chance that scientific breakthroughs resulting from these investments will be followed through into the actual development and production of vaccines that deliver health benefits, increasing the value of the original investment. Given these complementarities, which increase the cost-effectiveness of push funding, an advance market commitment might make donors and foundations more likely to want to increase resources flowing in to push funding.

Resources are finite. However, in the **short term,** there is no need for a sponsor making an advance market commitment to reduce other spending because:

- Making an advance market commitment has **no impact on government spending** measures (because payments will be measured only when the goods and services are delivered, even if the commitment is legally binding); in the United States, where the commitment would fall within the appropriations ceiling, we have proposed ways in which the commitment could be made without reducing the funds that are appropriated for other foreign assistance priorities.
- For **private foundations,** the commitment represents a claim on the foundation's assets, but does not directly reduce resources available for spending today. (Indeed, most private foundations would not

be able to reduce current spending, because of the rule that they must spend 5% of their principal each year.)[a]

In the **long term,** however, when a vaccine is developed, the commitment will clearly require the sponsors to make payments, using funds that could otherwise have been used elsewhere. To the extent that the commitment represents additional net spending, other lower priority spending will have to be reduced to accommodate this. However, the effect of the commitment on future budget allocations is likely to be considerably less than the headline $3 billion commitment, for three reasons:

- Sponsors would almost certainly spend significant sums buying a vaccine when it is developed anyway, even in the absence of making a commitment; this means the net cost of making a commitment is only the **additional price paid** under the guarantee compared with what would be charged without it.
- To the extent that the price paid initially under an advance market commitment is higher than donors normally pay for vaccines, the corollary is **permanently lower, sustainable vaccine prices more quickly,** as guaranteed by the producers under the advance market contract; thus the total future expected costs of buying vaccines may not be much higher than without a commitment; and their obligation will be strictly limited, unlike the present situation.
- The rapid development, production and distribution of vaccines would be likely to **save considerable costs elsewhere in development budgets** (such as purchasing of drugs, health care costs, R&D on these diseases), further reducing the net costs to donors.

This means that, while there is a long-term cost to the commitment that will have to be accommodated

---

Box 7.1 (continued)
Is there a budgetary tradeoff?

within future spending plans, the size of the additional spending that has to be accommodated as a result of the commitment is much less than it first appears. Depending on the nature of the donor's other spending plans and commitments, the net effect on the donor's budget in the future may be quite small. Furthermore, as shown in chapter 5, the expenditure to which the sponsor is committed is highly cost-effective, saving millions of lives at very low cost.

In conclusion, one of the attractive features of an

advance market commitment for potential sponsors is that there is no cash outlay until a vaccine is developed and used. This means that, in the short term, there is no direct budgetary pressure to reduce other spending when a commitment is made. On the contrary, a commitment would enhance the cost-effectiveness of current government and philanthropic funding by facilitating the more active engagement of the private sector, and by helping to turn research findings into useful products.

a. This is not true of public charities—which have a diverse funding base—such as the Vaccine Fund.

---

is a recognition that there might be a middle-income market. Moreover, funders could, if they choose, make it a condition of their grants that they receive a portion of intellectual property royalties received by institutions they fund. This is an area that merits further analysis than was possible within the context of the Working Group.

Regulatory and procurement systems

Existing procurement systems

Current procurement and regulatory systems for developing world vaccines depend heavily, though not exclusively, on the WHO and UNICEF. While some large countries—such as China, India and Indonesia—produce and buy their own vaccines, UNICEF and the Pan American Health Organization (PAHO) Revolving Fund are the primary agents of vaccine procurement for developing countries. And for Vaccine Fund–eligible countries, UNICEF is the largest global procurement system.

UNICEF and the Revolving Fund purchase only vaccines that are "pre-qualified" by the WHO, the official body advising UN agencies on the suitability of specific vaccine products for purchase.[4] Not only do UN agencies purchase only products on the WHO pre-qualified list, but many countries in the developing world also use it as a basis for their own product licensing and selection.

UNICEF supplies vaccines to 40% of the world's children. It works with governments to estimate needs for specific vaccines and immunization supplies, based on existing immunization program coverage, birth rates, expected availability of funds and other factors. It then aggregates those estimates over countries for each type of product and issues tenders through an international competitive bidding process. In negotiating with suppliers, factors taken into account include prices and a firm's track record for quality and reliability; when possible, UNICEF also considers different suppliers of the same product, to maintain a competitive supply environment.

On the financing side, UNICEF maintains accounts that are funded by individual donors, such as bilateral aid agencies, as well as national governments. It then matches the available funding for a given country to the products procured. UNICEF facilitates delivery of products in-country, with UNICEF staff often helping to ensure that the products make it safely through customs and to appropriate storage depots.

In 2002 UNICEF purchased $220 million worth of vaccines for use in 100 countries, representing 2 billion doses of vaccines.[5] The UNICEF procurement process has six steps: the decision to purchase a vaccine, development of specifications, identification of products meeting specifications (through WHO prequalification), publication of the tender, the adjudication and award process and receipt and release of the vaccine products.

Most of the countries of Latin America and the Caribbean procure their vaccines through the PAHO Revolving Fund, which began operation in 1979, to ensure a reliable supply of vaccines for the region's immunization programs.

PAHO in-country Expanded Programme of Immunization (EPI) advisors work with staff of the national immunization program to prepare orders on a periodic basis for specific vaccines and immunization supplies. Those requests are then aggregated at PAHO headquarters, which prepares tenders, negotiates prices, delivery dates and other contractual obligations and executes contracts. Payment is made to suppliers from the Revolving Fund. Then, when the products are delivered in-country, countries repay the Revolving Fund so that it is replenished for the next procurement round.

The Revolving Fund has been effective in coordinating procurement, increasing certainty for manufacturers and reducing prices. The number of countries participating has grown from 19 in 1979 to 34 in 2003; and the capitalization of the fund has grown from the original $1 million in 1979 to $20 million in 2003.

The need for long-term contracting

During our discussions, it became clear that industry attaches a great deal of importance to the further development and widespread use of binding, enforceable, long-term contracts for vaccines for developing countries.

UNICEF's usual procurement award for most commodities is a "long-term arrangement." Under a long-term arrangement, UNICEF and manufacturers agree to the commercial terms for products, such as prices, delivery schedules and packing requirements, so that when an order is placed, it can be delivered rapidly. Past long-term arrangements have typically had a duration of one to two years, but they can last as long as five years. UNICEF also provides the vaccine industry with forecasts for vaccine requirements (in three- or four-year increments), but these are indicative only (that is, they do not form an enforceable contract).

The challenge UNICEF faces is compounded by the fact that it is buying vaccines for 100 countries each year and that it is constrained by public sector purchasing regulations. The procurement decision for such a large number of countries, and making up such a large part of the market, creates a different relationship between buyer and sellers than would a procurement contract for a single country.

During our industry consultations, the point was made repeatedly and forcefully that the lack of binding contracts, and particularly binding long-term contracts, makes it difficult for potential suppliers to invest in long-term productive capacity, which would increase supply, permit greater reliability of supply and reduce the price. The result is higher prices for developing countries, lower use and occasionally supply constraints.

Aware of this concern, UNICEF has moved toward longer contracts where possible. But it appears that UNICEF is constrained in its ability to sign multiyear purchase agreements because its funding streams are typically guaranteed annually. In a recent procurement, the Vaccine Fund was able to give UNICEF multiyear funding "in trust" to support a multiyear contract. This arrangement involved setting aside money for future payments.

Donors and UNICEF need to work together to establish whether there is some way to enable UNICEF to enter long-term contracts, either by amending the rules governing UNICEF's financial position or by finding other possible financing mechanisms, such as underwriting agreements or promissory notes.

This situation also highlights the urgent need for reliable demand forecasts. Initiatives like the Accelerated Development and Introduction Plans for pneumococcus and rotavirus vaccines are attempting to recognize the pivotal importance of having an accurate forecast of demand. Improving accuracy in this area would be an important contribution to reducing risk for all parties.

Regulatory and procurement implications of advance market commitments

The existing system of regulation and procurement should be able to accommodate the existence of an advance market commitment with little or no adaptation.

The draft contract requires the supplier to obtain and maintain authorizations and approvals necessary to market and sell approved vaccines in the eligible countries, and to maintain appropriate qualification. It will be the responsibility of the Independent Adjudication Committee to determine whether a supplier of a qualifying product meets these conditions and is eligible for the price guarantee. In practice, the Independent Adjudication Committee would be expected to draw on the respected expertise of the WHO both to designate approved regulatory bodies for the purposes of the contract (or more likely to designate the WHO to approve regulatory bodies) and to require WHO prequalification as a condition of eligibility to supply the vaccine under the contract. However, though the Independent Adjudication Committee would in practice want to rely on the existing capacity and expertise of the WHO, it would retain the final decision about whether a supplier met the conditions for the guarantee.

The price guarantee contract would provide top-up payments; these could be used in support of procurements made through UNICEF, the PAHO Revolving Fund or other qualified buyers supplying the public sector in eligible countries. Although, as discussed above, there might be advantages in these bodies being able to make more use of long-term contracting, it is not strictly necessary for the implementation of an advance market commitment that these purchasers be able to do so. The reason for this is that the predictability of the advance market commitment is created by the Guarantee Agreement between the sponsors and the supplier, which guarantees sponsor co-payments, not by the terms of the actual procurement of vaccine.

While it is possible that some technical adjustment of existing procurement arrangements might be necessary to enable the main public sector buyers to buy the vaccines that are eligible for the advance market commitment, in principle the introduction of guaranteed co-payment envisaged by the advance market commitment should not cause any substantive difficulties for existing procurement processes.

Where to read more

- For updated information about the advance market commitment, please visit the Center for Global Development Making Markets for Vaccines website at www.cgdev.org/vaccine. This website also has links to other resources.

- For an easy-to-use spreadsheet model to calculate estimates of cost-effectiveness and total revenues for malaria, HIV and tuberculosis, please visit www.cgdev.org/vaccine.

- For a more detailed explanation of the theory underlying the advance market commitment, see Kremer, M. and R. Glennerster. 2004. *Strong Medicine: Creating Incentives for Pharmaceutical Research on Neglected Diseases.* Princeton, N.J.: Princeton University Press.

- For a more thorough discussion of some of the design issues for an advance market commitment, see Berndt, E. and J. Hurvitz. Forthcoming. "Vaccine Advance Purchase Agreements for Low-income Countries: Practical Issues." *Health Affairs.*

- For a detailed explanation of the estimates of cost-effectiveness and overall costs of an advance market commitment, see Berndt, E., R. Glennerster, M. Kremer, J. Lee, R. Levine, G. Weizsacker and H. Williams. 2005. "Advance Purchase Commitments for a Malaria Vaccine: Estimating Costs and Cost Effectiveness." Center for Global Development, Washington, D.C., available at www.cgdev.org/vaccine.

Notes

Summary

1. Though most of this report is concerned with vaccines, the discussion in this section also applies to R&D in drugs and diagnostic tools. We use the term "medicines" to mean drugs and vaccines.

2. Global Forum for Health Research (2004a).

3. Known in the jargon as product development public-private partnerships, or PDPPPs.

4. We have coined the term "advance market commitment" to distinguish this proposal from a commitment that guarantees firms sales in advance.

Chapter 1

1. Against diphtheria-tetanus-pertussis (DTP combinations), measles-mumps-rubella (MMR) and polio.

2. Measles Initiative (2005).

3. *Haemophilus influenzae* type B.

4. About $3 per dose for products that combine Hib with other antigens.

5. Davey (2002).

6. The Bacille Calmette–Guérin (BCG) vaccine protects against meningitis and disseminated tuberculosis. It has existed for 80 years and is widely used. However, it does not prevent primary infection and, more importantly, does not prevent reactivation of latent primary infection, the main source of bacillary spread in the community. The impact of BCG vaccination on transmission of *Myobacterium tuberculosis* is therefore limited. The World Health Organization (2004a) says, "the development of efficient, safe and affordable vaccines against TB [tuberculosis] must remain a global priority."

7. DTwP coverage in OECD countries has fallen from 90% to 34% as they now use DtaP (diphtheria, tetanus and acellular pertussis)—a more costly product that is thought to have a marginally better safety record and a more reliable production profile.

8. CVI Forum (1999), p. 6.

9. DiMasi, Hansen and Grabowski (2003).

10. Mercer Management Consulting (2002).

11. GAVI (2005b).

12. WHO (2003a).

13. Batson (2001).

14. Marketletter (2002).

15. Economists call this a problem of "time inconsistency" because the best policy to pursue changes over time, in a way that can be anticipated at the outset. Predicting a future change in policy, economic actors adjust their behavior today. It is typically solved by some form of institutional pre-commitment that prevents the authorities from "re-optimizing" in the later phase. An advance market commitment would provide such a commitment in this case.

16. Pecoul and others (1999), p. 364. Two of 13 are updated versions of previous products; two are the result of military research; and five come from veterinary research.

Chapter 2

1. We define "commercial investment" as investment by the for-profit sector, in the expectation of commercial returns.

2. Ernst and Young LLP (2000), p. 47.

3. Widdus and White (2004).

4. Michaud and Murray (1996).

5. Global Forum for Health Research (2004b).

6. Joint Economic Committee (2000).

7. NIH (2001).

8. PhRMA (2005).

9. National Science Foundation (2003).

10. Department of Defense (2004), p. 42.

11. Pecoul and others (1999), p. 364. Two of 13 are updated versions of previous products; 2 are the result of military research; and 5 come from veterinary research.

12. Acemoglu and Linn (2004).

13. See the MVI website www.malariavaccine.org for details.

14. See the IAVI website www.iavi.org for details.

15. See the Aeras website www.aeras.org/spotlight/gates829.html for details.

16. Sander and Widdus (2004).

17. DiMasi, Hansen and Grabowski (2003).

18. Malaria Vaccine Initiative (2004).

19. For example, these diseases include Huntington's disease, myoclonus, ALS (Lou Gehrig's disease), Tourette syndrome and muscular dystrophy.

20. Lichtenberg and Waldfogel (2003).

21. Henkel (1999).

22. Details of the procurement of a meningococcal C vaccine were provided in private communications by Angeline Nanni, formerly with Baxter and now with GAVI's Pneumo ADIP, and with David Salisbury, Principal Medical Officer of U.K.'s Department of Health.

23. Finkelstein (2003, 2004).

24. A caveat is that sales of this intranasal flu vaccine have been lower than expected, likely at least in part due to a high pricing strategy by the manufacturer.

25. Note that this is not guaranteed purchase of any particular product but a guarantee of funds available for qualified products.

26. IFPMA (2004).

Chapter 3

1. Some pull proposals, such as wildcard patent extensions or full patent buyouts, involve winner-take-all prizes. Academic literature on pull proposals has highlighted the difficulty with this approach. The main arguments are set out in chapter 4.

2. Clinical trials in developing countries are needed to ensure that a vaccine is safe and effective against the strains of the disease prevalent in the region.

3. Acemoglu and Linn (2004).

4. See the MVI website www.malariavaccine.org.

5. These estimates are somewhat controversial. See McCarthy, Wolf and Wu (1999) and Gallup and Sachs (2000).

6. Van de Perre and Dedet (2004).

7. The vaccine was originally developed in 1983 by the Walter Reed Army Institute of Research.

8. See the Rotavirus Vaccine Program website www.rotavirusvaccine.org.

9. Rotashield, the world's first rotavirus vaccine, was licensed for use in the United States in 1998. Prior to licensing, clinical trials in the United States, Finland and Venezuela had found it to be 80–100% effective at preventing severe rotavirus diarrhea, and researchers had detected no statistically significant serious adverse effects. But Wyeth, the manufacturer of Rotashield, withdrew the vaccine from the market in 1999, after it was discovered that it might have contributed to an increased risk of intussusception, or bowel obstruction, in 1 of every 12,000 vaccinated infants (CNN 2004).

10. See the ADIP website www.pneumoadip.org.

11. Apart from the modest cost for the institutional arrangements—that is, the cost of the Independent Adjudication Committee.

Chapter 4

1. *Force majeure* is a standard contracting clause that declares the contract null and void—and neither party liable for damages—if unforeseeable events fundamentally change the landscape in which the contract was written.

Chapter 5

1. Acemoglu and Linn (2004).

2. Grabowski, Vernon and DiMasi (2002) note that this is a comprehensive sample of the new chemical entities originating from and developed by the pharmaceutical industry that were introduced into the United States in 1990–94. Due to data limitations, we are unable to address whether the sales revenues of this

sample of self-originated new chemical entities is a representative sample of the sales revenues of all commercial pharmaceutical products. Sales revenue data from a larger sample of products are available from (for example) IMS Health or Scott Levin Associates. Further work could examine this and other potential sources of larger samples of sales revenue data.

3. Berndt and others (2005). Note that Grabowski, Vernon and DiMasi (2002) use this sales revenue data in combination with estimates of the cost of pharmaceutical development in order to estimate total returns; we did not use these cost of development estimates (nor any other cost of development estimates) in our analysis. The $3.1 billion figure reflects an assumed industry-wide cost of capital (that is, earnings foregone on other investment opportunities) of 8% (close to the annual average return on the stock market) and a downward adjustment of 10% for lower marketing expenditures. Rosenthal and others (2002) estimate that marketing expenditures relative to sales have remained relatively constant at 15%; however, promotion/sales ratios are lower globally, and this 15% figure is also partly the result of an accounting nuance where the values of free samples given to physicians are assessed at average retail price rather than manufacturing price. Hence a 10% reduction for marketing expenditures seems appropriate.

4. Berndt and others (2005). We project a total market of $750 million in net present value of revenues (2004) dollars in high- and middle-income countries. This estimate is based on annual purchases of malaria prophylaxis drugs, as presumably people would be willing to pay comparable amounts for a malaria vaccine as for malaria prophylaxis drugs. An estimate from the popular press (Reuters 2003) and correspondence with Pfizer suggest the annual market for malaria prophylaxis drugs from sales to travelers and tourists from developed countries and the military could be as much as $200 million, but others cite much lower figures. If a vaccine captured $100 million in peak sales and the profile of sales over time followed that of the average product in the Grabowski, Vernon and DiMasi (2002) sample, the total net present value of those sales would be about $750.7 million (assuming an 8% cost of capital). Adding in $100 million of additional revenues from private sales in low- and middle-income countries yields a default of $850 million in net present value of revenues outside the commitment program.

5. It is a coincidence that the $15 cost per DALY is the same as the $15 price per course of treatment.

6. Berndt and others (2005).

Chapter 6

1. Acemoglu and Linn (2004).

Chapter 7

1. Financial Reporting Standard 12 Provisions, Contingent Liabilities and Contingent Assets, September 1998.

2. Glennerster and Kremer (2000).

3. IDA terms are a 10-year grace period, a 0% interest rate, and maturities of 35 or 40 years.

4. The exception to this is if no product in a given category has been prequalified.

5. UNICEF (2002).

References

Acemoglu, D. and J. Linn. 2004. "Market Size in Innovation: Theory and Evidence from the Pharmaceutical Industry." *Quarterly Journal of Economics* 119 (3): 1049–90.

Asian Development Bank. 2001. *Immunization Financing in Developing Countries and the International Vaccine Market: Trends and Issues.* Manila, Philippines. [Accessed March 23, 2005, from www.adb.org/Documents/Books/Immuniza-tion_Financing/immunization_financing.pdf].

Batson, A. 2001. "Understanding the Vaccine Market and Its Economics." Presentation to the Out of the Box Group, July 26. [Accessed March 23, 2005, from www.vaccinealliance. org/site_repository/resources/21VacMarket.pdf].

Batson, A., S. Glass and E. Seiguer. 2003. "Economics of Vaccines: From Vaccine Candidate to Commercialized Project." In B. Bloom and P.H. Lambert, eds., *The Vaccine Book.* San Diego, Calif.: Elsevier Press.

Berndt, E., R. Glennerster, M. Kremer, J. Lee, R. Levine, G. Weizsacker and H. Williams. 2005. "Advance Purchase Commitments for a Malaria Vaccine: Estimating Costs and Cost Effectiveness." Center for Global Development, Washington, D.C. [Accessed March 23, 2005, from www.cgdev. org/vaccine].

Biotechnology Industry Association. 2003. BIO Testimony on Project BIOShield. Testimony before the House Energy and commerce Subcommittee on Health and the House Select Committee on Homeland Security Subcommittee on Emergency Preparedness and Response Regarding Project Bioshield Act of 2003, March 27, Washington, D.C. [Accessed March 23, 2005, from www.bio.org/healthcare/ biodefense/20030327.asp].

Bloom, D. and D. Canning. 2000. "The Health and Wealth of Nations." *Science* 287: 1207–09.

Bloom, D., D. Canning and P. Malaney. 2000. "Demographic Change and Economic Growth in East Asia." *Population and Development Review* 26 (suppl.): 257–90.

Brown, P. 2000. "The Invisible Culprit." *GAVI Immunization Focus* August: 4–6. [Accessed March 23, 2005, from www. vaccinealliance.org/resources/aug2000.pdf].

Cairncross, S. and V. Valdmanis. 2004. "Disease Control Priorities Project." Working Paper 28. National Institutes of Health, Fogarty International Center, Bethesda, Md.

Capell, K. 2004. "Vaccinating the World's Poor." *Business Week,* April 26. [Accessed March 23, 2005, from www.businessweek. com/magazine/content/04_17/b3880098.htm].

Centers for Disease Control and Prevention. 2003. "Global Progress Toward Universal Childhood Hepatitis B Vaccination." *Morbidity and Mortality Weekly Report* 52 (36): 868–70.

Children's Vaccine Initiative. 1999. "A Plethora of Hi-tech Vaccines: Genetic, Edible, Sugar Glass, and More." *CVI Forum.* July (18): 5–24. [www.vaccinealliance.org/resources/ cvi_18e.pdf].

CNN. 2004. "Rotavirus Vaccine Reenters Market after Ban." May 4.

Creese, A., K. Floyd, A. Alban and L. Guinness. 2002. "Cost-effectiveness of HIV/AIDS interventions in Africa: a Systematic Review of the Evidence." *The Lancet* 359 (9318): 1635–42. [Accessed March 23, 2005, from www.ncbi.nlm. nih.gov/entrez/query.fcgi?cmd=Retrieve&db=pubmed& dopt=Abstract&list_uids=12020523].

Davey, S. 2002. *State of the World's Vaccines and Immunization.* Geneva: World Health Organization. [Accessed March 23, 2005, from www.eldis.org/static/DOC13001.htm].

DiMasi, J., R. Hansen and H. Grabowski. 2003. "The Price of Innovation: New Estimates of Drug Development Costs." *Journal of Health Economics* 22 (2): 151–330.

Economist, The. 2004. "A Worrying Failure to Engage the Drug Industry in the War on Terror." April 22.

Ernst and Young LLP. 2000. *Convergence: Biotechnology Industry Report, Millennium Edition.* New York.

Finkelstein, A. 2003. *Health Policy and Technological Change: Evidence from the Vaccine Industry.* NBER Working Paper 9460. Cambridge, Mass.: National Bureau of Economic Research.

————. 2004. "Static and Dynamic Effects of Health Policy: Evidence from the Vaccine Industry." *Quarterly Journal of Economics* 119 (2): 527–64. [Accessed March 23, 2005, from www.nber.org/~afinkels/papers/VaccinesJan04.pdf].

Forbes, A. 2000. "Microbicides 2000: Unclogging the Research Pipeline." *HIV InSite Spotlight Report,* March 23. [Accessed March 23, 2005, from www.lifelube.org/research/forbes-microbicides-2000.html].

Fraser, C. 2004. "An Uncertain Call to Arms." *Science* 304: 359.

Gallup, J. L. and J. D. Sachs. 2000. "The Economic Burden of Malaria." CID Working Paper 52. Harvard University, Center for International Development, Cambridge, Mass.

GAVI (Global Alliance for Vaccines and Immunization). 2004. "Annual Deaths in 2002 from Vaccine-Preventable Diseases: WHO Estimates." Geneva. [www.vaccinealliance.org/General_Information/Immunization_informa/Diseases_Vaccines/vaccine_preventable_deaths.php].

————. 2005a. "Disease Information: Pneumococcus." Geneva. [www.vaccinealliance.org/General_Information/Immunization_informa/Diseases_Vaccines/pneumo.php].

————. 2005b. "Fact Sheet: The Global Alliance for Vaccines and Immunization (GAVI) and the Vaccine Fund." Geneva. [http://gavi.elca-services.com/resources/FS_GAVI_and_Vaccine_Fund_en_Jan05.pdf].

Glass, S. N., A. Batson and R. Levine. 2001. "Issues Paper: Accelerating New Vaccines." Global Alliance for Vaccinves and Immunization, Financing Task Force, Geneva. [Accessed March 23, 2005, from www.gaviftf.org/forum/pdf_cd/18IssuesPaper.pdf].

Glennerster, R. and M. Kremer. 2000. "A World Bank Vaccine Commitment." Policy Brief 57. Brookings Institution, Washington, D.C. [Accessed March 23, 2005, from www.brookings.edu/comm/policybriefs/pb57.htm].

Global Forum for Health Research. 2004a. *10/90 Report on Health Research.* Geneva. [www.globalforumhealth.org/site/002__What%20we%20do/005__Publications/001__10%2090%20reports.php].

————. 2004b. *Monitoring Financial Flows for Health Research.* Geneva. [www.globalforumhealth.org/site/002__What%20we%20do/005__Publications/004__Resource%20flows.php].

Grabowski, H. G., J. Vernon and J. A. DiMasi. 2002. "Returns on Research and Development for 1990s New Drug Introductions." *PharmacoEconomics* 20 (suppl. 3): 11–29.

Hanson, K., N. Kikumbih, J. Armstrong Schellenberg, H. Mponda, R. Nathan, S. Lake, A. Mills, M. Tanner and C. Lengeler. 2003. "Cost-effectiveness of Social Marketing of Insecticide-treated Nets for Malaria Control in the United Republic of Tanzania." *Bulletin of the World Health Organization* 81 (4): 269–76.

Henkel, J. 1999. "Orphan Drug Law Matures into Medical Mainstay." *FDA Consumer,* May/June.

Hollis, A. 2005. "An Efficient RewardSystem for Pharmaceutical Innovation." University of Calgary, Department of Economics. [Accessed March 23, 2005, from http://econ.ucalgary.ca/fac-files/ah/drugprizes.pdf].

Hsu, J. C., and E. S. Schwartz. 2003. *A Model of R&D Valuation and the Design of Research Incentives.* NBER Working Paper w10041. Cambridge, Mass.: National Bureau of Economic Research.

Hubbard, T. and J. Love. 2004. "A New Trade Framework for Global Healthcare R&D." *PLoS Biology* 2 (2): 147–50. [Accessed March 23, 2005, from www.plosbiology.org/archive/1545-7885/2/2/pdf/10.1371_journal.pbio.0020052-L.pdf].

IAVI (International AIDS Vaccine Initiative). 2000. "Presidential Council on AIDS Prioritizes Accelerated Vaccine Development." New York. [www.iavi.org/viewfile.cfm?fid=841].

IFPMA (International Federation of Pharmaceutical Manufacturers and Associations). 2004. "The Pharmaceutical Innovation Platform: Sustaining Better Health for Patients Worldwide." Geneva.

Institute of Medicine. 2003. *Financing Vaccines in the 21st Century: Assuring Access and Availability.* Washington, D.C.: The National Academies Press.

Joint Economic Committee. 2000. "The Benefits of Medical Research and the Role of the NIH." Washington, D.C.

Kaddar, M., P. Lydon and R. Levine 2004. "Financial Challenges of Immunization: a Look at GAVI." *Bulletin of the World Health Organization* 89 (2): 697–702.

Klausner, R. D., A. S. Fauci, L. Corey, G. J. Nabel, H. Gayle, S. Berkley, B. F. Haynes, D. Baltimore, C. Collins, R. G. Douglas, J. Esparza, D. P. Francis, N. K. Ganguly, J. L. Gerberding, M. I. Johnston, M .D. Kazatchkine, A. J. McMichael, M. W. Makgoba, G. Pantaleo, P. Piot, Y. Shao, E. Tramont, H. Varmus and J. N. Wasserheit. 2003. "The Need for a Global HIV Vaccine Enterprise." *Science* 300: 2036–39. [www.aidscience.org/Science/Science--Klausner_et_al_300(5628)2036.htm].

Kremer, M. 2000a. *Creating Markets for New Vaccines Part I: Rationale.* NBER Working Paper w7716. Cambridge, Mass.: National Bureau of Economic Research.

————. 2000b. *Creating Markets for New Vaccines Part II: Design Issues.* NBER Working Paper w7717. Cambridge, Mass.: National Bureau of Economic Research.

Kremer, M. and R. Glennerster. 2004. *Strong Medicine: Creating Incentives for Pharmaceutical Research on Neglected Diseases.* Princeton, N.J.: Princeton University Press.

LaForce, F. M. 2003. "Defeating the Scourge of Meningococcal Disease in Africa: A Work in Progress." Meningitis Vaccine Project, Ferney-Voltaire, France. [Accessed March 23, 2005, from www.meningvax.org/files/essay-fmlaforce-0311.pdf].

Lanjouw, J. 2003. "Drug Patents: Taking the Poorest Out of the Fight." University of California, Berkeley, Agricultural and Resource Economics Department. [http://are.berkeley.edu/~lanjouw/milken.pdf].

Levine, R., M. Kinder and the What Works Working Group. 2004. *Millions Saved: Proven Successes in Global Health.* Center for Global Development, Washington, D.C.

Lichtenberg, F. R. and J. Waldfogel. 2003. *Does Misery Love Company? Evidence from Pharmaceutical Markets Before and After the Orphan Drug Act.* NBER Working Paper w9750. Cambridge, Mass.: National Bureau of Economic Research,

Mabey, D., R. Peeling and M. Perkins. 2001. "Rapid and Simple Point of Care Diagnostics for STIs." *Sexually Transmitted Infections* 77: 397–398. [Accessed March 23, 2005, from http://sti.bmjjournals.com/cgi/content/extract/77/6/397].

Madrid, Yvette. 2001. *A New Access Paradigm: Public Sector Actions to Assure Swift, Global Access to AIDS Vaccines.* New York: International AIDS Vaccine Initiative. [Accessed March 23, 2005, from www.iaen.org/files.cgi/387_publicsector.pdf].

Malaria Vaccine Initiative. 2004. "Malaria Vaccine R&D: The Case for Greater Resources." Bethesda, Md. [www.malariavaccine.org/files/Two-page-funding.pdf].

Mallaby, S. 2004. "Opening the Gates." *The Washington Post.* April 5.

Marketletter. 2002. "Double-Digit Growth Rates Elude Most Blockbuster Firms, Says Datamonitor." May 27. Quoted in Institute of Medicine. 2003. *Financing Vaccines in the 21st Century: Assuring Access and Availability.* Washington, D.C.: National Academies Press.

McCarthy, F. D., H. Wolf and Y. Wu. 1999. *The Growth Costs of Malaria.* NBER Working Paper 7541. Cambridge, Mass.: National Bureau of Economic Research.

Measles Initiative. 2005. "Fast Facts." [Accessed March 23, 2005, from www.measlesinitiative.org/facts2.asp].

Mercer Management Consulting. 2002. "Lessons Learned: New Procurement Strategies for Vaccines." Final report to the GAVI Board. New York. [Accessed March 23, 2005, from http://gaviftf.info/docs_activities/pdf/lessons_learned_draft_final.pdf].

Michaud, C. and C. J. L. Murray. 1996. "Resources for Health Research and Development in 1992: A Global Overview." In *Investing in Health Research and Development: Report of the Ad Hoc Committee on Health Research Relating to Future Intervention Options.* Geneva: World Health Organization.

Moree, M. 2003. "Malaria Vaccine R&D." Malaria Vaccine Initiative, Bethesda, Md. [Accessed March 23, 2005, from www.malariavaccine.org/files/Moreefinal.pdf].

Murray, C. and A. Lopez. 1996. *Global Burden of Disease.* Cambridge, Mass.: Harvard University Press.

———. 1997a. "Alternative Projections of Mortality and Disability by Cause 1990–2020: Global Burden of Disease Study." *The Lancet* 349: 1498–504.

———. 1997b. "Global Mortality, Disability, and the Contribution of Risk Factors: Global Burden of Disease Study." *The Lancet* 349: 1436–42.

———. 1997c. "Mortality by Cause for Eight Regions of the World: Global Burden of Disease Study." *The Lancet* 349: 1269–76.

National Institute of Allergy and Infectious Diseases. 2000. "Drug Development." Summit on Development of Infectious Disease Therapeutics, September 26–27, Bethesda, Md. [Accessed March 23, 2005, from www.niaid.nih.gov/dmid/drug/summit.htm].

National Science Foundation. 2003. *Research and Development in Industry.* Washington, D.C.

NIH (National Institutes of Health). 2001. "A Plan to Ensure Taxpayers' Interests Are Protected." NIH Response to the Conference Report Request for a Plan to Ensure Taxpayers' Interests are Protected. Bethesda, Md. [Accessed February 2005, from www.nih.gov/news/070101wyden.htm].

Nordhaus, W. 2003. "The Health of Nations: The Contribution of Improved Health to Living Standards." In Kevin H. Murphy and Robert H. Topel, eds., *Measuring the Gains from Medical Research: An Economic Approach.* Chicago, Ill.: University of Chicago Press.

Pecoul, B., P. Chirac, P. Trouiller and J. Pinel. 1999. "Access to Essential Drugs in Poor Countries." *Journal of the American Medical Association* 281 (4): 361–67.

PhRMA (Pharmaceutical Research and Manufacturers of America). 2005. *Pharmaceutical Industry Profile 2005.* Washington, D.C.: PhRMA.

Progressive Health Partners. 2000. "Current U.S. Legislative and Administration Proposals: Supporting and AIDS Vaccine." Prepared for the International AIDS Vaccine Initiative. Washington, D.C. [Accessed March 23, 2005, from http://phpartners.com/pubs/currentproposalsreport.pdf].

Reuters. 2003. "Pfizer Announces Potential Malaria Discovery." June 17.

Rosenthal, M. B., E. R. Berndt, J. M. Donohue, R. G. Frank and A. M. Epstein. 2002. "Promotion of Prescription Drugs to Consumers." *New England Journal of Medicine* 346 (7): 498–505.

Rotavirus Vaccine Program. 2005. "Rotavirus Facts." [Accessed March 23, 2005, www.rotavirusvaccine.org/rotavirus-facts.htm].

Sander, A. and R. Widdus. 2004. "The Emerging Landscape of Public-Private Partnerships for Product Development." Initiative on Public-Private Partnerships for Health, Geneva.

UNICEF (United Nations Children's Fund). 2002. *UNICEF Supply Division Annual Report 2002.* New York. [Accessed March 23, 2005, from www.unicef.org/supply/supply_division_annual_report2002.pdf].

United States Department of Defense. 2004. *Strategies to Leverage Research Funding: Guiding DOD's Peer Reviewed Medical Research Programs.* Washington, D.C.: The National Academies Press.

United States Food and Drug Administration. 1983. "The Orphan Drug Act (as amended)." Washington, D.C. [Accessed March 23, 2005, from www.fda.gov/orphan/oda.htm].

University of California Atlas of Global Inequity. "Cause of Death." University of California, Santa Cruz, Center for Global, International and Regional Studies. [Accessed March 23, 2005, from http://ucatlas.ucsc.edu/cause.php].

Van de Perre, P. and J.-P. Dedet. 2004. "Vaccine Efficacy: Winning a Battle (Not War) Against Malaria." *The Lancet* 364 (9443): 1380–83.

WHO (World Health Organization). 2003a. "Investing in Health: a Summary of the Findings of the Commission on Macroeconomics and Health." CMH Support Unit. Geneva. [Accessed March 23, 2005, from http://www3.who.int/whosis/cmh].

———. 2003b. "Progress Towards Global Immunization Goals: Summary Presentation of Key Indicators." Geneva. [Accessed March 23, 2005, from www.who.int/vaccines-surveillance/documents/SlidesGlobalImmunization_7_%20May_2002.ppt].

———. 2003c. *The World Health Report 2003: Shaping the Future.* Geneva. [Accessed March 23, 2005, from www.who.int/whr/2003/chapter4/en/].

———. 2004a. "BCG Vaccine." *Weekly Epidemiological Record* 4 (79): 27–38. [Accessed March 23, 2005, from www.who.int/wer/2004/en/wer7904.pdf].

———. 2004b. "Vaccines, Immunizations, and Biologicals, Immunization Profile—United States of America." Geneva. [Accessed March 23, 2005, from www.who.int/vaccines/globalsummary/immunization/countryprofileselect.cfm].

———. 2004c. *WHO Vaccine-Preventable Diseases: Monitoring System.* Geneva. [Accessed March 23, 2005, from www.who.int/vaccines-documents/GlobalSummary/GlobalSummary.pdf].

———. 2004d. "World Report on Knowledge for Better Health." Geneva. [Accessed March 23, 2005, from www.who.int/rpc/meetings/en/WR2004AnnotatedOutline.pdf].

Widdus, R. 2000. "AIDS Vaccines for the World: Preparing Now to Assure Access." International AIDS Vaccine Initiative, New York. [Accessed March 23, 2005, from www.iavi.org/pdf/accessblueprint.pdf].

Widdus, R. and K. White. 2004. "Combating Diseases Associated with Poverty: Financing Strategies for Product Development and Potential Role of Public-Private Patnerships (Abridged Version)." Initiative on Public-Private Partnerships for Health. Presented at Combating Diseases Associated with Poverty, April 15–16, London.

Wittet, S. 2001. "Hepatitis B Vaccine Introduction: Lessons Learned in Adovcacy, Communication and Training." Occasional Paper 4. Children's Vaccine Program, Seattle, Wash. [Accessed March 23, 2005, from www.childrensvaccine.com/files/CVP_Occ_Paper4.pdf].

World Bank. 1993. *World Development Report 1993: Investing in Health.* Washington, D.C.

———. 2003. *World Development Indicators 2003.* Washington, D.C.

World Bank, Bill & Melinda Gates Foundation and GAVI (Global Alliance for Vaccines and Immunization). 2002. *Accelerated Introduction of Priority New Vaccines in Developing Countries—From Credible Investment Case to Accelerated Development and Introduction Plan (ADIP).* New York: McKinsey and Company. [Accessed March 23, 2005, from www.gaviftf.info/docs_activities/pdf/GAVI_workshop_McKinsey_presentation.pdf].

Appendix A

Abbreviations

ACIP	Advisory Committee on Immunization Practices
ADIP	Accelerated Development and Introduction Plans
AIDS	acquired immunodeficiency syndrome
BCG	Bacille Calmette–Guérin—a vaccine for tuberculosis
BIO	Biotech Industry Organization
CDC	Centers for Disease Control and Prevention
CEA	Council of Economic Advisors
CVI	Children's Vaccine Initiative
DALY	disability-adjusted life year
DFID	Department for International Development
DNDi	Drugs for Neglected Diseases Initiative
DTaP	diphtheria, tetanus and acellular pertussis
DTP	diphtheria, tetanus and pertussis
DTwP	diphtheria, tetanus and whole-cell pertussis
EMVI	European Malaria Vaccine Initiative
EPI	Expanded Programme on Immunization
FDA	Food and Drug Administration
FRS	Federal Reporting Standard
GAVI	Global Alliance for Vaccines and Immunization
GDP	gross domestic product
GMP	Global Microbicide Project
GNP	gross national product
HepB	hepatitis B
HHVI	Human Hookworm Vaccine Initiative
Hib	haemophilus influenzae type B
HIV	human immunodeficiency virus
IAC	Independent Adjudication Committee
IAVI	International AIDS Vaccine Initiative
IDA	International Development Association
IFF	International Financing Facility
IFFIm	International Finance Facility for Immunization
IFPMA	International Federation of Pharmaceutical Manufacturers and Associations
IMCI	Integrated Management of Childhood Illness
IOWH	Institute for OneWorld Health
IPM	International Partnership for Microbicides
IPR	intellectual property rights
MDP	Microbicide Development Project
MMV	Medicines for Malaria Venture
MVI	Malaria Vaccine Initiative
NIAID	National Institute of Allergy and Infectious Diseases
NIH	National Institutes of Health
OPV	oral polio vaccine
PDPPPs	product development public-private partnerships
PDVI	Pediatric Dengue Vaccine Initiative
PhRMA	Pharmaceutical Research and Manufacturers of America
R&D	research and development
SAAVI	South African AIDS Vaccine Initiative
U.K.	United Kingdom
U.S.	United States
UN	United Nations
UNICEF	United Nations Children's Fund
USAID	United States Agency for International Development
VFC	Vaccines for Children
WHO	World Health Organization

Objectives of the Working Group

The Advance Market Commitment (originally "Pull Mechanisms") Working Group is a policy research group convened by the Global Health Policy Research Network at the Center for Global Development to explore the feasibility of advance guarantee agreements as a tool for stimulating research, development and production of vaccines for neglected developing-country diseases. Funding for Working Group meetings, analytic work and consultations was provided under a grant from the Bill & Melinda Gates Foundation.

Because the power and limitations of push mechanisms are reasonably well understood, the Working Group has focused exclusively on whether and how to put into operation advance guarantees as an *additional* new tool for global health products. The results of this work are intended primarily to inform the donor community, which may wish to move toward implementation of such an arrangement as one of several instruments to improve access to affordable vaccines for the developing world.

The Working Group was convened solely for the purpose of exploring the practicality and value of advance contracting; it does not have and will not seek the legal status, the budget or the mandate to implement such an agreement. Members of the Working Group were selected for their knowledge and expertise, and participate on a voluntary basis in their individual capacities.

We focused exclusively on vaccines in this Working Group for a number of reasons. First, vaccines are among the most cost-effective of health interventions, and immunization programs have been shown to be enormously successful. Second, a key constraint to even greater effectiveness of immunization programs is availability of and access to new products related to the specific needs of children in the developing world. And finally, vaccines are purchased mainly by the public sector and development of new vaccines is a global public good so it is appropriate for donors to be thinking about the most effective ways to channel their immunization funds. We did not choose vaccines because it is the only area where advance contracting would work—many of the principles outlined in this report may be transferable to drugs or diagnostics with some modifications.

Although the Working Group is not expected to continue after the publication of this report, resources related to the group's work will be available at the Center for Global Development's website (www.cgdev.org/vaccine).

Profiles of Working Group members

Abhijit Banerjee, Massachusetts Institute of Technology

Abhijit Banerjee is the Ford Foundation Professor of Economics in the Department of Economics at Massachusetts Institute of Technology, the Director of the Poverty Action Lab and the ex-President of the Bureau for Research in Economic Analysis and Development. Previously, he taught at Princeton University and Harvard University before joining the Massachusetts Institute of Technology faculty in 1996. He received the Malcolm Adeshesiah Award in 2001 and the Mahalanobis Memorial Medal in 2000. He is a member of the Governing Council of the Econometric Society and the American Academy of Arts and Sciences, and he has been a Guggenheim Fellow and Alfred P. Sloan Research Fellow. His areas of research are development economics, the economics of financial markets and the macroeconomics of developing countries.

Amie Batson, World Bank

Amie Batson is a Senior Health Specialist in the Health, Nutrition and Population unit of the World Bank. She is also the co-chair of the Financing Task Force of the Global Alliance for Vaccine and Immunization charged with supporting governments and international partners to improve sustainable financing, and exploring innovative financing mechanisms to accelerate the development and introduction of priority vaccines in the developing world. Prior to joining the World Bank, she was a joint World Health Organization/United Nations Children's Fund staff member in the Global Programme for Vaccines. She led the work on public-private partnerships for vaccines, launching a new relationship and strategies based on the underlying economics of manufacturing.

Ernst Berndt, Massachusetts Institute of Technology

Ernst Berndt is the Louis B. Seley Professor of Applied Economics at the Massachusetts Institute of Technology's Sloan School of Management. He also is co-director of the Harvard–Massachusetts Institute of Technology Health Sciences and Technology Biomedical Enterprise Program and directs the National Bureau of Economic Research Program on Technological Progress and Productivity Measurements.

Lael Brainard, Brookings Institution

Lael Brainard is Founding Director of the Poverty and Global Economy Initiative at the Brookings Institution, where she holds the New Century Chair in International Economics. She served as Deputy National Economic Adviser and Chair of the Deputy Secretaries Committee on International Economics during U.S. President Bill Clinton's administration. As the U.S. "Sherpa" to the G-7/G-8, she is credited with shaping the 2000 G-8 Development Summit, which included developing country leaders for the first time and laid the foundations for the Global Fund to Fight AIDS, Tuberculosis and Malaria. Before coming to Washington, she served as Associate Professor of Applied Economics at the Massachusetts Institute of Technology's Sloan School of Management. Previously, she worked at McKinsey and Company advising clients on strategic challenges. She is the recipient of a White House Fellowship and a Council on Foreign Relations International Affairs Fellowship, and a member of the Council on Foreign Relations and the Board of Wesleyan University.

David Cutler, Harvard University

David Cutler is Associate Dean of Social Sciences and Professor of Economics in the Department of Economics and Kennedy School of Government at Harvard University. He served on the Council of Economic Advisers and the National Economic Council during U.S. President Bill Clinton's administration and advised the presidential campaigns of Bill Bradley and John Kerry. Among other affiliations, he has held positions with the National Institutes of Health and the National Academy of Sciences. Currently, he is a Research Associate at the National Bureau of Economic

Research and a member of the Institute of Medicine. He is the author of *Your Money or Your Life: Strong Medicine for America's Health Care System.*

David Gold, Global Health Strategies

David Gold is an attorney and principal of Global Health Strategies. Most recently, he was Vice President for Policy and Public Support at the International AIDS Vaccine Initiative, where he oversaw the creation of its global policy and advocacy programs, as well as its regional programs in North America, Europe, Japan and Latin America. He is also co-founder of the AIDS Vaccine Advocacy Coalition, a consumer-based organization that advocates for AIDS vaccine development and delivery. From 1991–95 he headed the Medical Information Program at Gay Men's Health Crisis, the world's first and largest AIDS organization, and edited its newsletter on HIV therapies, *Treatment Issues.* He has also served on research advisory panels for a number of different organizations including the World Health Organization, the United Nations, the U.S. National Institutes of Health and a number of pharmaceutical companies.

Peter Hutt, Covington & Burling

Peter Barton Hutt is a senior counsel in the Washington, D.C., law firm of Covington & Burling, specializing in food and drug law and teaches Food and Drug Law each winter term at Harvard Law School. He is the co-author of *Food and Drug Law: Cases and Materials,* and was Chief Counsel for the Food and Drug Administration from 1971 to 1975. He is a member of the Institute of Medicine of the National Academy of Sciences, has served on the Institute of Medicine Executive Committee, and other National Academy of Sciences and Institute of Medicine committees. He serves on the Panel on the Administrative Restructuring of the National Institutes of Health. He serves on a wide variety of academic and scientific advisory boards and on the Board of Directors of venture capital startup companies.

Randall Kroszner, University of Chicago

Randall S. Kroszner is Professor of Economics at the Graduate School of Business of the University of Chicago. He is Editor of the *Journal of Law and Economics* and Associate Director of the George J. Stigler Center for the Study of the Economy and the State. He also is a Faculty Research Fellow of the National Bureau of Economic Research and a Visiting Scholar at the American Enterprise Institute. He served as a Senate-confirmed member of the President's Council of Economic Advisers from 2001 to 2003. While on the council, he was involved in policy formulation for a wide range of domestic and international issues, including the Millennium Challenge Account and economic growth and development. He has served as a consultant to the International Monetary Fund, the World Bank, the Inter-American Development Bank, the Swedish Finance Ministry, the Board of Governors of the Federal Reserve System and several Federal Reserve Banks, and currently serves as a Research Consultant for the Federal Reserve Bank of Chicago. He has been a visiting professor at the Stockholm School of Economics, the Free University of Berlin and the Institute for International Economic Studies at the University of Stockholm. His research interests include corporate governance, conflicts on interest in financial services firms, banking and financial regulation, debt restructuring and forgiveness, international financial crises and political economy.

Thomas McGuire, Harvard University

Thomas McGuire is Professor of Health Economics in the Department of Health Care Policy at Harvard Medical School. His research focuses on the design and impact of health care payment systems, the economics of health care disparities and the economics of mental health policy. He has contributed to the theory of physician, hospital and health plan payment. His current research includes application of theoretical and empirical methods from labor economics to the area of health care disparities. For more than 25 years, he has conducted academic and policy research on the economics of mental health. He is a member of the Institute of Medicine, and a co-editor of the *Journal of Health Economics.*

Tomas Philipson, U.S. Food and Drug Administration

Tomas Philipson is a professor in the Harris School of Public Policy at the University of Chicago and a faculty member in the Department of Economics and the Law School. His research focuses on health economics. During 2003/04, he served as the Senior Economic Advisor to the Commissioner of the Food and Drug Administration and currently serves as the Senior Economic Advisor to the Administrator of the Centers for Medicare and Medicaid Services. Previously, he was a visiting faculty member at Yale University and a visiting fellow at the World Bank in the winter of 2003. He is a co-editor of the journal *RAND Forums in Health Economics* of Berkeley Electronic Press and is affiliated with a number of professional organizations, including the National Bureau of Economic Research, the George J. Stigler Center for the Study of the Economy and the State, the Robert Wood Johnson Clinical Scholars Program, the Northwestern/University of Chicago Joint Center for Poverty Research, the National Opinion Research Center and the American Economic Association.

Leighton Read, Alloy Ventures

Leighton Read is a General Partner at Alloy Ventures, following 14 years as a biotechnology entrepreneur and investor. He co-founded Affymax NV and founded Aviron, a biopharmaceutical company focused on vaccines for infectious disease, where he served as Chairman and CEO until 1999 and Director until its acquisition by MedImmune in 2002. He was also a partner in Interhealth Limited, an investment partnership. He is a director of Avidia, Alexza and Cambrios Technologies and has served as director for a number of other biotechnology companies and on the executive committee of the Biotechnology Industry Organization. He has

also won several awards as co-inventor of technology underlying the Affymetrix GeneChip™.

Tom Scholar, International Monetary Fund

Tom Scholar is the United Kingdom Executive Director to the International Monetary Fund and the World Bank. He also serves as Minister (Economic) at the British Embassy, Washington. Previously, he was Economic Adviser to the H.M. Treasury and Principal Private Secretary to the Chancellor of the Exchequer at the H.M. Treasury.

Rajiv Shah, Bill & Melinda Gates Foundation

Rajiv Shah is the deputy director for Strategic Opportunities and Evaluation at the Bill & Melinda Gates Foundation. Previously, he managed the global health program's policy and finance portfolio, helped manage the program's largest grant effort, the Vaccine Fund, and shaped overall strategy for engaging with bilateral and multilateral financial institutions. He served as the health care policy advisor on the Gore 2000 presidential campaign in Nashville, Tennessee, and on Philadelphia Mayor John Street's New Century Committee. He started, managed and sold a health care consulting firm, Health Systems Analytics, which served clients including some of the largest health systems in the country. In 1995 he co-founded Project IMPACT, an award-winning national nonprofit that conducts leadership, mentoring, media and political activism activities.

David Stephens, Emory University

David Stephens is Professor of Medicine, Microbiology and Immunology and Epidemiology; Director, Division of Infectious Diseases, Department of Medicine; and Executive Vice Chair of the Department of Medicine, Emory University School of Medicine, and holds the Stephen W. Schwarzman Distinguished Professorship in Internal Medicine at Emory University. He has contributed to the development of meningococcal, pneumococcal and *Bacillus anthracis* vaccines including efforts to develop a meningococcal conjugate vaccine that is affordable for countries in Sub-Saharan Africa. He has also helped lead efforts to address vaccines for biodefense and emerging infections serving as the Executive Director of the Centers for Disease Control and Prevention–sponsored Southeastern Center for Emerging Biological Threats, as the Emory Principal Investigator for the National Institutes of Health–sponsored Southeastern Research Center of Excellence in Biodefense and Emerging Infections and as director of a National Institutes of Health–sponsored new pathway center at Emory for interdisciplinary research in vaccinology. He is a past chair of the Food and Drug Administration's National Vaccine Advisory Committee and has more than 200 publications in infectious diseases, molecular pathogenesis, vaccines and epidemiology.

Wendy Taylor, BIO Ventures for Global Health

Wendy Taylor is the Executive Director of BIO Ventures for Global Health. Previously, she was the Director of Regulatory Affairs and Bioethics for the Biotechnology Industry Organization (BIO) where she spearheaded BIO's global health initiative. Joining BIO in November 2001, she negotiated on behalf of the biotech industry the third reauthorization of the Prescription Drug User Fee Act with the Food and Drug Administration; established and led BIO's Regulatory Affairs Committee and worked with the Food and Drug Administration to address a range of regulatory issues important to the biotech industry. She also has extensive experience in the executive and legislative branches of the U.S. government, including positions at the Office of Management and Budget, the U.S. Department of Health and Human Services and the U.S. House Committee on Ways and Means.

Adrian Towse, Office of Health Economics

Adrian Towse is the Director of the Office of Health Economics. He is a Visiting Professor at the University of York and a Non-executive Director of the Oxford Radcliffe Hospitals NHS Trust, one of the United Kingdom's largest hospitals. His current research interests include the use of "risk-sharing" arrangements between health care payers and pharmaceutical companies; the economics of pharmacogenetics; economic issues around access to, and R&D for the development of, treatments for less developed country diseases; the economics of medical negligence; and measuring productivity in health care.

Sean Tunis, U.S. Department of Health and Human Services

Sean Tunis is currently the Director of the Office of Clinical Standards and Quality and Chief Medical Officer at the Centers for Medicare and Medicaid Services. He oversees several major elements of the Centers for Medicare and Medicaid Services quality and clinical policy portfolio, including the development of national coverage policies and quality standards for Medicare and Medicaid providers, and serves as a senior advisor to the administrator on clinical and scientific policy. Previously, he was a senior research scientist with the Lewin Group, Director of the Health Program at the Congressional Office of Technology Assessment and a health policy advisor to the U.S. Senate Committee on Labor and Human Resources. He holds an adjunct faculty position in the Department of Medicine at the Johns Hopkins School of Medicine, and continues to practice as a part-time emergency room physician in Baltimore, Md.

Sharon White, U.K. Department for International Development

Sharon White is presently Director of Policy at the U.K. Department for International Development. Previously she held a series of other posts in the United Kingdom and international public sector including senior economist in the Poverty Reduction Group of the World Bank, adviser to Prime Minister Tony Blair on

U.K. welfare reform and First Secretary (Economic) at the U.K. Embassy to the United States.

Victor Zonana, Global Health Strategies

Victor Zonana is principal and co-founder of Global Health Strategies. Previously, he was founding Vice President for Communications of the Vaccine Fund and Vice President for Communications of the International AIDS Vaccine Initiative between 1998 and 2001. During the first five years of U.S. President Bill Clinton's administration, he served as Deputy Assistant Secretary for Public Affairs of the Department for Health and Human Services. Before joining the government, he was a journalist for *The Wall Street Journal* and *The Los Angeles Times*. He was the 1990 winner of the John Hancock award for distinguished financial journalism and was nominated twice for a Pulitzer Prize.

Staff

Owen Barder, Center for Global Development

Owen Barder is a Senior Program Associate at the Center for Global Development. He has previously worked in the U.K. Treasury, No. 10 Downing Street, the U.K. Department for International Development and the South African Treasury.

Gargee Ghosh, Bill & Melinda Gates Foundation

Gargee Ghosh is a Program Officer and Economist with the Bill & Melinda Gates Foundation, where she works primarily on innovative financing and delivery for vaccines and immunization. She helps manage the foundation's work with the Global Alliance for Vaccines and Immunization, and particularly its funding arm the Vaccine Fund. Prior to joining the foundation, she worked with the Center for Global Development's Global

Health Policy Research Network as the project manager for its Pull Mechanisms Working Group. She also spent several years as a management consultant with McKinsey and Company in New York and London working with the firm's health care and nonprofit clients around the world.

Co-chairs

Alice Albright, Vaccine Fund

Alice Albright is Vice President and Chief Financial Officer of the Vaccine Fund. Previously, she worked in international financial markets with an emphasis on emerging markets. From 1999 to 2001, she was a Principal in the Leveraged Buy-Out practice of the Carlyle Group in Washington, D.C. She was a Vice President at JP Morgan from 1989 to 1999 where she held various positions in the emerging markets, corporate finance, credit portfolio management and lending areas. From 1987 to 1989, she was an Associate in Bankers Trust's Latin American Merchant Bank. From 1985 to 1987, she worked as a management consultant at Citicorp, conducting financial management assignments in Latin America and Europe. She is a Chartered Financial Analyst.

Michael Kremer, Harvard University

Michael Kremer is the Gates Professor of Developing Societies in the Department of Economics at Harvard University and Senior Fellow at the Brookings Institution. He is a Fellow of the American Academy of Arts and Sciences and a recipient of a MacArthur Fellowship and a Presidential Faculty Fellowship. His recent research examines education and health in developing countries, immigration and globalization. He and Rachel Glennerster recently published *Strong Medicine: Creating Incentives for Pharmaceutical Research on Neglected Diseases.* His articles have been published in journals including the *American Economic Review, Econometrica* and the *Quarterly Journal of Economics.* He previously served as a teacher in Kenya. He founded and was the first executive director of WorldTeach, a nonprofit organization that places more than 200 volunteer teachers annually in developing countries (1986–89).

Ruth Levine, Center for Global Development

Ruth Levine, Senior Fellow and Director of Programs at the Center for Global Development, is a health economist with 14 years' experience in health and family planning financing issues in Latin America, eastern Africa, the Middle East and South Asia. She currently leads the Center's Global Health Policy Research Network and is principal staff on the Millennium Project Education and Gender Equality Task Force. Before joining the Center for Global Development, she designed, supervised and evaluated health-sector loans at the World Bank and the Inter-American Development Bank. She also conducted research on the health sector and led the World Bank's knowledge management activities in the area of health economics and finance between 1999 and 2002. Since 2000, she has worked with the Financing Task Force of the Global Alliance on Vaccines and Immunization. Between 1997 and 1999, she served as the adviser on the social sectors in the Office of the Executive Vice President of the Inter-American Development Bank. She is co-author of *The Health of Women in Latin America and the Caribbean* and *Millions Saved: Proven Successes in Global Health.*

Individuals consulted

During the course of this project, many individuals offered comments, critiques and suggestions. These individuals are listed below, but bear no responsibility for the content or recommendations of this report. We apologize for any omissions.

- Pedro Alonso, Scientific Director, Manhica Health Centre, Manhica, Mozambique and Head, Center for International Health, University of Barcelona, Spain
- Bill Antholis, German Marshall Fund U.S.
- John Audley, German Marshall Fund U.S.
- Ripley Ballou, Clinical R&D, GlaxoSmithKline Biologicals, Rixensart, Belgium
- Luis Barreto, Aventis-Pasteur
- Carolyn Bartholomew, then Chief of Staff for Congresswoman Nancy Pelosi
- Simon Best, Ardana
- Alan Brooks, Program for Accessible Technologies in Health
- Graham Brown, Department of Medicine, University of Melbourne, Australia
- Josh Buger, Vertex
- Chip Cale, GSK Biologicals
- Sandra Chang, Tropical Medicine and Medical Microbiology, University of Hawaii
- Rob Chess, Nectar Therapeutics
- Chris Collins, Joint United Nations Programme on HIV/AIDS
- Tim Cooke, Mojave Therapeutics
- Martinho Dgedge, Expanded Program on Immunization Manager, Mozambique
- Carter Diggs, Senior Technical Advisor, U.S. Agency for International Development
- Steve Drew, GSK Biologicals
- Laura Efros, Merck Vaccine Division
- Thomas Egwang, MedBiotech Laboratories, Uganda
- Ibrahim El Hassan, Institute of Endemic Diseases, University of Khartoum, Sudan
- Howard Engers, Armauer Hansen Research Institute, Ethiopia
- Elaine Esber, Merck Vaccine Division
- Sarah Ewart , Malaria Vaccine Initiative
- Andrew Farlow, University of Oxford
- David Fleming, then Centers for Disease Control and Prevention; now Bill & Melinda Gates Foundation
- Michael Fleming, Merck Vaccine Division
- Martin Friede, Initiative for Vaccine Research, World Health Organization
- Joel Friedman, Center for Budget Policy and Priorities
- Geno Germano, Wyeth
- Roger Glass, Centers for Disease Control and Prevention
- Michel Greco, formerly Aventis
- Shanelle Hall, United Nations Children's Fund, Supply Division
- Jane Haycock, U.K. Department for International Development
- Rob Hecht, then World Bank, now International AIDS Vaccine Initiative
- Russell Howard, Maxygen
- Suresh Jadhav, Serum Institute
- Stephen Jarrett, United Nations Children's Fund, Supply Division
- Soren Jepsen, European Malaria Vaccine Initiative, Copenhagen, Denmark
- Miloud Kaddar, World Health Organization
- Cheikh Kane, J P Morgan
- Hannah Kettler, Bill & Melinda Gates Foundation
- Marie-Paule Kieny, Director, Initiative for Vaccine Research, World Health Organization
- Wenceslaus Kilama, African Malaria Vaccine Testing Network, Tanzania

- Fred Kironde, Makerere University, Kampala, Uganda
- Andrew Kitua, Director General, National Institute for Medical Research, Tanzania
- Richard Kogan, Center for Budget Policy and Priorities
- Antoniana Krettli, Fiocruz, Brazil
- James Kublin, Merck Vaccine Division
- Steve Landry, Bill & Melinda Gates Foundation
- Odile Leroy, Clinical and Regulatory Affairs, European Malaria Vaccine Initiative
- Orin Levine, Pneumococcal Accelerated Development and Introduction Plan
- Clem Lewin, Chiron
- Adel Mahmoud, Merck Vaccine Division
- Frank Malinoski, Wyeth
- Kevin Marsh, Kenya Medical Research Institute, Kilifi, Kenya
- Sean McElligot, Merck Vaccine Division
- Eunice Miranda, GSK Biologicals
- Marge Mitchell, Merck Vaccine Division
- Melinda Moree. Malaria Vaccine Initiative
- Debbie Myers, GSK Biologicals
- Angeline Nanni, Pneumococcal ADIP
- Thomas Netzer, Merck Vaccine Division

- Tim Obara, Merck Vaccine Division
- Paul Offit, Childrens' Hospital of Philadelphia
- Stewart Parker, Targeted Genetics
- Jerry Parrot, Human Genome Sciences
- Alix Peterson Zwane, University of California, Berkeley
- Gina Rabinovich, Bill & Melinda Gates Foundation
- Patricia Roberts, Malaria Vaccine Initiative
- Una Ryan, Avant Theraputics Inc
- Jerry Sadoff, Aeras Global TB Vaccine Foundation
- Mark Sanyour, Merck Vaccine Division
- Andrew Segal, Genitrix
- Alan Shaw, Merck Vaccine Division
- Tim Sullivan, Princeton University Press
- Larry Summers, Harvard University
- Jim Tartaglia, Aventis-Pasteur
- Jean Tirole, Institut d'Economie Industrielle
- Thomas Vernon, Merck Vaccine Division
- John Wecker, Rotavirus ADIP
- Lowell Weiss, Bill & Melinda Gates Foundation
- Roy Widdus, Institute for Public Private Partnerships in Health
- Michel Zaffran, World Health Organization

Appendix E

A tool to estimate cost effectiveness of an advance market commitment

Michael Kremer and Rachel Glennerster, authors of the recent book *Strong Medicine: Creating Incentives for Pharmaceutical Research on Neglected Diseases,* set out the theoretical underpinnings of pull incentives in more detail. Ernst Berndt and others have developed a spreadsheet model (available for download from the Center for Global Development website at www.cgdev.org/vaccine) that allows users to manipulate all relevant variables in a flexible and user-friendly way, thereby permitting the analysis of a large number of different scenarios.

The spreadsheet allows for the analysis of costs and benefits of commitments for malaria, HIV and tuberculosis vaccines under various assumptions of vaccine characteristics as well as various contract parameters on the price and quantity of vaccines that would be purchased at the initial, high price. The spreadsheet combines these user-entered assumptions with a collection of demographic and disease burden data to estimate the cost per DALY saved as well as to calculate the net present value of the revenues that would accrue to a vaccine developer.

For example, the user may vary general parameters (such as the discount rate and the cost effectiveness threshold for a DALY), and parameters that define vaccine efficacy and the number of required doses. The user may change the set of countries covered by the program manually, by disease burden and/or using a GNP per capita cutoff. The user can also vary the conditions of adoption, including steady-state adoption rates and the length of time to reach the steady state. A technical guide posted online with the spreadsheet explains the calculations in detail in the order that the worksheets appear in the Microsoft Excel file. Since parameters can be modified and results displayed in the graphical user interface, the user will rarely, if ever, need to refer to these detailed sheets. Berndt and others (2005) discuss both the general results of the spreadsheet analysis and sensitivity checks.

Model term sheet for Framework Agreement

1. Parties:	One or more nongovernmental, grant-making organizations (such as a foundation) or governmental grant-making organizations (such as the U.S. Agency for International Development or the U.K. Department for International Development) (each, a **"Funder"**)[1] and one or more pharmaceutical or biotech companies[2] that will work within the Framework (as defined below) to develop eligible vaccine(s) (each, a **"Developer"**).
2. Purpose:	Create a legally binding series of agreements[3] that guarantees the developer(s) of a [____] vaccine[4] that meets the requirements set forth in the agreements a specific price for each qualified sale of the vaccine in certain designated developing countries (the **"Framework"**). The Framework Agreement will clearly state the goals and objectives of the Framework with regard to the target disease, the eligible countries and the affected populations.[5]
3. Benefits to Funder:	Fulfills the Funder's philanthropic mission (or a statutory or regulatory mandate, in the event Funder is a governmental organization) by giving Developers an economic incentive to (a) select and implement R&D projects that are likely to lead to vaccines developed specifically for diseases concentrated in developing countries, and (b) establish manufacturing capacity for production of such vaccines.
4. Benefits to Developers:	Establishes a specific price for all eligible sales of the vaccine in developing countries that allows the Designated Supplier (as defined below) to cover, over the term of the agreements, R&D costs as well as manufacturing costs and to make an acceptable return on its investment. The guaranteed price will be based on a per-patient dosing regimen to provide the required prophylactic benefit and will be paid on all eligible sales up to the maximum number specified in the Guarantee and Supply Agreement (the **"Maximum Guaranteed Amount"**). For example, if a course of 3 immunizations are required to provide the necessary immunity, the guaranteed price is $15 and the Maximum Guaranteed Amount is 200 million, then the Developer would receive the guaranteed price of $15 only upon an eligible sale of all three doses comprising the course of treatment. If the Developer's total eligible sales equal the Maximum Guaranteed Amount, 600 million doses, or 200 million courses of treatment, then the Developer would receive a total payment of $3 billion.[6]

Notes

1. The Framework Agreement and Guarantee Agreement term sheets were designed to accommodate a variety of Funders, despite the fact that there are substantial differences between governmental and nongovernmental organizations in areas such as funding capacity and ability to contractually commit to the Guarantee Agreement. We concluded that traditional commercial mechanisms for ensuring compliance, such as letters of credit or escrow arrangements, would be unattractive to potential Funders as they would result in increased transaction costs and unnecessarily tie up funds that could be made available for more immediate opportunities. Instead, we designed a bilateral contract structure, which would permit the Developer to pursue standard contract remedies, such as money damages and specific performance, if the Funders fail to satisfy their financial commitments.

2. The Framework and Guarantee term sheets were designed to allow participation by both pharmaceutical companies and biotechnology companies. We considered, but did not incorporate, an alternative funding system recommended by a few of the biotechnology companies interviewed that would provide for interim payments, upon the achievement of certain predetermined milestones, to create incentives for research and early-stage development activities and encourage venture capital investment in emerging companies committed to the Framework. We intend that intermediate incentives of this kind will be created by the commercial activities of Developers in the expectation of being remunerated through sales of vaccines under the Guarantee Agreement.

3. Initially, the Working Group considered establishing the Framework Agreement as a form of unilateral agreement. A unilateral agreement is an offer by one party, in this case the Funder, which only becomes a contract when it is accepted by the other party, the offeree or in this case the Developer.

A unilateral agreement permits the offeror is withdraw its offer prior to acceptance, and what constitutes acceptance is not always clear, particularly in this context. We thought this risk might create too much uncertainty for the Developer and thereby dilute the effect of the commitment. The Framework Agreement as reflected in this term sheet would be bilateral agreement, which would be binding on the Funders as soon as one or more Developers sign on.

4. The Working Group initially intended that the Framework Agreement and Guarantee Agreement term sheets would be used for both late-stage and early-stage vaccine candidates. However, on further consideration, we decided that a form approach did not make sense for late-stage vaccine candidates, given the fact that specific Developers and Approved Vaccines had been identified for Rotavirus, and the recognition that each Developer had specific needs and objectives. Instead, the Working Group recommended that the Developers and the Funders directly negotiate long-term supply or other appropriate arrangements to ensure reliable, affordable supply to meet the long-term needs of Eligible Countries, while providing appropriate rewards for the vaccine developer.

5. Each Framework Agreement will establish a specific price for qualified sales of an Approved Vaccine, by supplementing the "base price" paid by a vaccine purchaser (such as UNICEF on behalf of the developing country) up to a certain fixed amount.

6. We concluded that the price guarantee should be for "per course of treatment" rather than "per dose." This approach provides incentives to ensure that all doses of multiple dose vaccines are administered, and encourages the development of vaccines requiring fewer doses where scientifically possible.

5. **Principal Responsibilities of the Funder:**	The Funder shall (a) upon satisfaction of the conditions precedent set forth in Section 7, enter into a Guarantee and Supply Agreement (in the form attached to the Framework Agreement) with one or more Designated Supplier(s) (as defined below),[7] (b) fund the operation of the Independent Adjudication Committee (as defined below) in accordance with budgeted amounts, (c) indemnify the members of the Committee for claims and losses arising out of the performance of their duties under the Framework Agreement and the Guarantee and Supply Agreement,[8] (d) retain the Contract Administrators (as defined below) to administer the Framework in accordance with budgeted amounts, (e) maintain in strict confidence any confidential business information submitted to it by the Developers, and (f) agree to be bound by decisions of the Committee acting within the scope of its authority.
6. **Principal Responsibilities of Developers:**	Each Developer shall (a) provide confidential reports to the Independent Adjudication Committee on the progress of its development efforts at the times specified by the Committee (it is contemplated that these reports would be high-level annual status reports at the outset and would increase in frequency and detail as the development efforts advance),[9] (b) provide such technical information as may be reasonably requested by the Committee in order to confirm that the conditions precedent set forth in Section 7 have been satisfied, and (c) agree to be bound by decisions of the Committee acting within the scope of its authority.
7. **Conditions Precedent to Obligations of Funder:**	It shall be a condition precedent to Funder's obligation to enter into and perform its obligations under the Guarantee and Supply Agreement that the vaccine meet (a) the technical specifications outlined in Section 8 below, and (b) the usability requirements outlined in Section 9 below.[10]
8. **Technical Specifications:**	For a vaccine to meet the technical specifications it must, subject to Section 10, satisfy the approval, safety and efficacy requirements set forth in Schedule A.
9. **Usability Requirements:**	For a vaccine to meet the usability requirements it must, subject to Section 10, satisfy the dosage, means of delivery, storage, shelf life and other requirements set forth in Schedule A.
10. **Waiver of Conditions Precedent:**	After the effective date of the Framework Agreement the Independent Adjudication Committee may (by a 2/3 vote of its members or at the direction of the Funder) waive or modify the technical specifications or usability requirements in a way that does not materially increase the cost of performance for a Developer. For purposes of illustrating the foregoing, if a specification called for 60% effectiveness, the Committee could, by a 2/3 vote of its members, reduce the requirement to 50% effectiveness, but could not increase it to 70% effectiveness under this provision.[11]

7. Until a vaccine is approved under the conditions set forth in Section 7 of the Framework Agreement term sheet, the Funder is only required to commit to the Framework Agreement, and fund the functions of the Independent Adjudication Committee. Once an Approved Vaccine is identified, the Developer has the right, and the Funder the obligation, to enter into the Guarantee Agreement with respect to that product.

8. Indemnification was deemed to be particularly important to attract qualified members to serve on the Independent Adjudication Committee. It is contemplated that this indemnification would be similar to that which is provided to officers and directors of corporations. Accordingly, the indemnification of the members of the Independent Adjudication Committee may exclude intentional misconduct or actions that are conducted in bad faith or for personal gain.

9. Developers may provide confidential information to the Independent Adjudication Committee in two circumstances. First, Developers would submit progress reports to the Independent Adjudication Committee during the term of the Framework Agreement. These reports will provide a way to evaluate the effectiveness of the mechanism during the research and early development periods. These reports, if not promising, may permit the Funder to withdraw from the Framework Agreement under Section 25 of the term sheet.

Second, for those Developers seeking to participate at a later date, the Framework Agreement requires some evidence that the Developer has a technology or expertise with scientific promise for the development of an Approved Vaccine.

10. Although the Framework Agreement is designed to create an enforceable bilateral contract between the Developers and the Funders, the Funders would not be obligated to enter into the Guarantee Agreement until a product is tendered that meets certain minimum technical specifications, such as approval of both the product and its manufacturing process by a qualified regulatory body and certain safety, efficacy and use requirements.

11. Because there was concern that the Developer should be assured that the Funder could not change the rules of the game after the Framework Agreement was entered into, technical requirements cannot be changed to increase the burden of those requirements, unless there is a significant change in circumstances with respect to the disease that would significantly reduce the need for a vaccine or undermine the specifications, such as a dramatic decrease in disease prevalence, a significant change in disease transmission or progression or a major advancement in treatment. As noted below, these types of changes would be subject to judicial review. Technical requirements may be decreased, however, at the discretion of the Independent Adjudication Committee.

11. Testing and Acceptance:	The Developer shall submit the vaccine to the Independent Adjudication Committee for testing and acceptance. The Committee shall be responsible for making determinations with respect to whether a vaccine tendered by a Developer satisfies the conditions precedent set forth in Section 7, provided that the Independent Adjudication Committee shall have the right to delegate this responsibility to one or more third parties that it determines are qualified to make such determinations and are independent and unbiased, such as, for example, the World Health Organization's prequalification process.[12] Further, the Committee shall have the right to retain one or more consultants or rely on the actions of governmental or other third parties, such as the United States Food and Drug Administration, in making its determinations. In addition, the Committee shall have authority to grant waivers of, or make modifications to, the application of specific technical specifications or usability requirements as provided in Sections 10 and 22.
12. Designated Supplier:	If the Independent Adjudication Committee determines that the conditions precedent have been satisfied (or if the conditions that have not been satisfied are waived or modified), then (a) the vaccine submitted by the Developer to the Committee shall be deemed an **"Approved Vaccine,"** (b) the Developer of the Approved Vaccine shall be deemed a **"Designated Supplier,"** and (c) if requested by the Designated Supplier, the Funder shall enter into the Guarantee and Supply Agreement with the Designated Supplier within thirty (30) days of the date of the final, written determination of the Committee.[13]
13. Composition of Independent Adjudication Committee:	The Funder shall establish a committee (the **"Independent Adjudication Committee"** or the **"Committee"**), which shall comprise not less than [5] members. Members of the Committee will have expertise in the following fields: (a) immunization practices, (b) public health, (c) vaccinology and vaccine development, manufacturing and commercialization, (d) pediatric and internal medicine, (e) social and community attitudes on immunization, (f) economics, (g) contract law and (h) the vaccine industry, in each case, as applicable, with developing country perspectives. Members of the Committee shall serve a term of [_] years. Vacancies on the Committee will be filled by the remaining members of the Committee.
14. Actions of the Committee:	Each member of the Independent Adjudication Committee shall have one vote. Fifty percent of the members of the Committee, rounded up, shall constitute a quorum. Except as provided in Sections 10, 20 and 22, all decisions of the Committee shall be made by majority vote of the members at a meeting at which a quorum exists.

12. The Working Group recognized that it would be extremely
costly to create an Independent Adjudication Committee
that was fully capable of independently evaluating, approving
and monitoring the Approved Vaccines and their ongoing
production. Accordingly, the Framework Agreement permits the Independent Adjudication Committee to rely on
third parties and their procedures, such as the WHO and
its prequalification process.

13. As noted above, the Framework Agreement is designed to
be self-executing with respect to the Funders, providing the
Developers with the right to enter into the Guarantee Agreement on the terms specified in the Framework Agreement.
The Framework Agreement is also designed to permit more
than one Developer to receive funds under the Guarantee Agreement. For the reasons discussed in the Guarantee
Agreement, and more fully in the report, the Working Group
determined not to pursue a winner-takes-all approach.

15. Duties of the Committee: The Committee will (a) seek to identify independent, unbiased and expert-qualified institutions and procedures to assist with determining whether a product meets the technical specifications and usability requirements and that can provide ongoing review of product safety and efficacy and manufacturing, (b) if necessary, designate Approved Regulatory Countries and Approved Manufacturing Countries from time to time, (c) evaluate products presented by Developers to determine if they satisfy the conditions precedent, (d) at its discretion or at the direction of Funder, waive or modify the application of specific technical specifications or usability requirements pursuant to Section 10, (e) if requested or as necessary, conduct multiple bilateral or multilateral meetings with Developer(s) in order to provide information about testing and acceptance procedures, waivers and modifications to the conditions precedent, market demand and supply forecasting, disease epidemiology and other relevant information,[14] (f) using the standards specified in Schedule B, determine whether subsequent vaccines are superior to the original Approved Vaccine, whether for certain target populations, epidemiological conditions or otherwise, and designate new Approved Vaccine(s) and new Designated Supplier(s), (g) after an Approved Vaccine has been designated, monitor the sales and use of such Approved Vaccine for ongoing compliance with the technical specifications and usability requirements set forth in Sections 8 and 9 and decertify any vaccine that is not in material compliance with such specifications and requirements, and (h) determine whether the technical specifications and usability requirements set forth in Sections 8 and 9 or the Maximum Guaranteed Amount or Funder's other payment obligations under the Guarantee and Supply Agreement should be modified in whole or in part based on *force majeure* criteria pursuant to Section 22.

16. Duties of Committee Members: Each member of the Independent Adjudication Committee shall, in the exercise of its authority under the Framework Agreement, have the same fiduciary duties (including duty of care and duty of loyalty) as the director of a Delaware corporation.[15]

17. Contract Administrator: The Funder shall retain one or more individuals (each, a **"Contract Administrator"**) to implement the decisions of the Independent Adjudication Committee and to perform such other administrative, support and other tasks as may be assigned by the Committee, subject to the approved budget for administrative expenses.

18. Budget: The parties shall agree on a budgeting process to ensure that the reasonable expenses of the Independent Adjudication Committee and the Contract Administrators will be reimbursed by Funder.[16]

14. It is contemplated that the Developers would have the right to consult with the Independent Adjudication Committee, much the same way that companies consult with the FDA in the United States, to discuss the design of clinical trials, the structure of drug approval applications, the country or countries in which such approval will be sought, the possibility of granting waivers and other issues relating to the approval of an Approved Vaccine.

15. The duties of a corporate director under Delaware Law are the duty of loyalty, the duty of care and the duty of good faith. The duty of loyalty requires the director to place the corporation's interests above his or her own. The duty of care requires the director to act with certain minimum level of skill and deliberation. The duty of good faith requires that a director not act with bad faith, or engage in intentional misconduct.

16. A Funder's obligation to reimburse the Independent Adjudication Committee is subject to the requirement that its expenses be reasonable. A Funder may want to give further consideration to mechanisms that would permit it to regulate the cost of the Independent Adjudication Committee without compromising the Independent Adjudication Committee's independence.

19. Addition of New Developers to the Framework:	During the period beginning on the effective date of the Framework Agreement and ending [36] months thereafter, one or more entities may become parties to the Framework Agreement (*i.e.*, Developers) upon written acceptance of the terms of the Framework Agreement by such entity. Thereafter, additional entities may become parties to the Framework Agreement upon (a) written approval by the Committee if the new entity has technology or expertise that shows promise for the development of an Approved Vaccine, and (b) written acceptance of the terms of the Framework Agreement by the new entity; provided that no entity may become a party to the Framework Agreement with respect to a product after it commenced clinical trials for such product without the consent of the Funder.[17]
20. Addition of New Designated Suppliers:	The Independent Adjudication Committee may (by a 2/3 vote of its members and using the standards specified in Schedule B) determine that a newly developed vaccine satisfies the conditions precedent in Section 7, subject to its waiver and modification authority, and is superior to the previously selected Approved Vaccine, whether for certain target populations or epidemiological conditions or otherwise. Upon such a determination by the Committee, the Developer of the newly developed vaccine shall have the right to become a party to the Guarantee and Supply Agreement, whereupon the Developer of the new vaccine shall be deemed a "Designated Supplier" and the new vaccine shall be deemed an "Approved Vaccine." The addition of new Designated Suppliers and Approved Vaccines shall, in each case, be subject to the original Maximum Guaranteed Amount set forth in the Guarantee and Supply Agreement.[18]
21. Reserved Rights of Developer:	Developer reserves all rights, and the Framework shall not apply, to sales of any Approved Vaccine (a) outside the eligible countries identified in the Guarantee and Supply Agreement, and (b) in the military or travelers markets.
22. Force Majeure	In the event that there is a substantial change in circumstances with respect to [disease] in the countries identified in the Guarantee and Supply Agreement, including, without limitation, its incidence, its characteristics or methods for its treatment or prevention, such that the technical specifications outlined in Section 8, or the usability requirements outlined in Section 9 no longer achieve the original objectives, the Committee shall have the right (by a 3/4 vote of its members), using the criteria set forth in Schedule C, to (a) modify the technical specifications or the usability requirements, as applicable, (b) reduce the Maximum Guaranteed Amount or the Funder's other financial obligations to reflect changes in the number of eligible countries or the incidence of untreated [disease] in those countries, or (c) terminate the Framework Agreement. Unlike other decisions of the Committee, these decisions shall be subject to judicial review by an appropriate forum to determine whether the Committee abused its discretion.[19]
23. Representation and Warranties:	[TBD]

17. These procedures were intended to strike a balance between, on the one hand, permitting companies with promising technology or relevant expertise to participate in the Framework and, on the other hand, discouraging free riders who would operate outside the Framework and sign on only at the last minute. If companies do not sign on to the Framework, the agreement would lose its binding effect. Moreover, it would be difficult for the Funders to monitor the success of the Framework, particularly with respect to research and early development, without the periodic reporting by the Developer required under the Framework Agreement. Funders may wish to strike a different balance, such as allowing companies to join the Framework up until they commence pivotal trials.

18. The Working Group devoted considerable discussion to the question of whether more than one Developer would be permitted to receive payments under the Guarantee Agreement. On the one hand, the Working Group felt that it was important to preserve incentives for product improvements and that it would be important to use superior products should they be developed. On the other hand, the Working Group was concerned companies might be less willing to risk large investments in early research if they faced the prospect of entry of "me too" products offering no significant advance over the original vaccine. However, many of the industry participants interviewed by the Working Group indicated that they would prefer to have multiple suppliers over a winner-takes-all approach. Recognizing that independent research may lead to the development of substantially similar products, another option would be to permit any qualifying vaccines, whether or not superior, that are tendered within a window (*e.g.,* one year) after the approval of the initial Approved Vaccine to be accepted without showing superiority, provided that the second vaccine resulted from independent research and is not simply a generic copy.

19. The Framework Agreement for an early stage vaccine could be in force for a decade or more before a vaccine candidate is presented for final review to the Independent Adjudication Committee. Accordingly, a force majeure provision permitting the Funder to alter the Framework Agreement based upon extraordinary events has been included. The force majeure clause would void or alter the Framework Agreement in the event of major changes to technology, disease epidemiology or the like that make a vaccine either inappropriate or unnecessary or that would require a change in the specifications that would be more burdensome to the Developers. These determinations are subject to judicial review.

24. Indemnification and Insurance:	[TBD]
25. Term and Termination:	The term will begin on the date that [__] Developers have executed the Framework Agreement (the "Effective Date") and, unless earlier terminated pursuant to Section 22 or this Section 25, continue until the [_____] anniversary of that date, unless a Guarantee and Supply Agreement has been entered into prior to such anniversary in which case the term shall continue until the later of such anniversary and the expiration or earlier termination of the Guarantee and Supply Agreement.
	Funder shall have the right to terminate the Framework Agreement (a) after the [_____] anniversary of the Effective Date if no Developer has commenced GLP toxicology studies for a product that shows reasonable promise to become an Approved Vaccine, (b) after the [_____] anniversary of the Effective Date if no Developer has commenced clinical trials for a product that shows reasonable promise to become an Approved Vaccine, (c) after the [_____] anniversary of the Effective Date if no Developer has commenced a pivotal clinical trial designed to demonstrate that a product meets the technical specifications and the usability requirements for an Approved Vaccine, (d) after the [_____] anniversary of the Effective Date if no Developer has filed an NDA or other comparable filing for a product that meets the technical specifications and the usability requirements for an Approved Vaccine, and (e) after the [_____] anniversary of the Effective Date if no Developer has entered into a Guarantee and Supply Agreement with respect to an Approved Vaccine.[20]
26. Remedies in the Event of Breach:	[TBD]
27. Dispute Resolution:	[Arbitration under AAA rules in NY, NY].
28. Governing Law:	[New York law].
29. Waiver of Immunity:	If the Funder is a sovereign, it will (a) acknowledge that the transactions are subject to private commercial law, and (b) if it has not already done so, waive sovereign immunity.
30. Other Provisions:	Other covenants, terms and provisions as requested by legal counsel to Funder or the Developers.
31. Exhibits:	Guarantee and Supply Agreement.

20. The Funders have the right to terminate the Framework Agreement if certain interim milestones have not been achieved in a timely manner. This provision is included to provide the Funders with an option to end the agreement if the Framework does not appear to be stimulating productive research and development activities. This would permit Funders to pursue other, more promising opportunities.

Schedule A to model term sheet for Framework Agreement (Malaria)

Note that these specifications were developed for example purposes only. Further analyses and consultations would be required to arrive at the appropriate specifications for the actual guarantee.

I. Technical requirements

A. Indication:
1. Prevention of clinical episodes of Plasmodium falciparum malaria in infants and young children.

B. Target population:
1. 0–4-year-olds in areas of malaria transmission in Africa.

C. Efficacy requirements
1. Prevent at least 50% of clinical episodes of malaria due to P. falciparum.

D. Duration of Protection
1. At least 24 months with no qualitative or quantitative exacerbation of subsequent disease.

E. Interference
1. No interference with other pediatric vaccines.

F. Regulatory Approval and Quality Control
1. Regulatory approval of a product, with labeling that meets or exceeds the other technical specifications and usability requirements set forth herein, in one or more of Canada, France, Germany, Italy, Japan, [Mexico], Spain, the United Kingdom, the United States, [others] and such other countries with regulatory standards and procedures that are at least equivalent to those in the foregoing countries, as the Independent Adjudication Committee may designate from time to time (each, an **"Approved Regulatory Country"**). The Committee shall have the right to remove any Approved Regulatory Country if its regulatory standards and procedures change after the effective date of the Framework Agreement or the date that it was approved by the Committee, as applicable.

2. Manufacture of product in one or more of Canada, France, Germany, Italy, Japan, [Mexico], Spain, the United Kingdom, the United States, [others] and such other WHO-qualified countries with regulatory standards and procedures that are at least equivalent to those in the foregoing countries, as the Independent Adjudication Committee may designate from time to time (each, an **"Approved Manufacturing Country"**). The Committee shall have the right to remove any Approved Manufacturing Country if its regulatory standards and procedures change after the effective date of the Framework Agreement or the date that it was approved by the Committee, as applicable.

3. In lieu of one or both of the foregoing requirements, the Committee may rely on an independent, unbiased, expert third party (*e.g.*, the WHO) to determine that the product meets or exceeds the other technical specifications and usability requirements set forth herein, and to ensure that the facilities where, and conditions under which, the product is manufactured are in compliance with Good Manufacturing Practices and other applicable international standards with respect to the manufacture, holding and shipment of vaccines, in each case throughout the term of the Guarantee and Supply Agreement.

II. Usability requirements

A. Dosage:
1. 1 to a maximum of 4 immunizations; EPI schedule preferred.

B. Route of immunization:
1. Any, provided conducive to use on a large scale in Eligible Countries as defined in the Guarantee and Supply Agreement.

C. Presentation:
1. Multi-dose vials.

D. Storage
1. TBD.
2. TBD, e.g. Two years shelf life.

E. Safety Requirements
TBD, consistent with existing practices by UNICEF and PAHO.

Schedule B to model term sheet for Framework Agreement (Malaria)

Standards and Criteria

1. Standards for Addition of New Designated Suppliers
   TBD.
2. Criteria for Termination of Funder's Payment Obligations
   TBD.

Model term sheet for
Guarantee and Supply Agreement

1. Parties:	Funder(s) and one or more Designated Suppliers.[1]
2. Purpose:	Guarantee that the Designated Supplier(s) receive a specific price[2] for each sale of the Approved Vaccine[3] if the sale qualifies as a Qualified Sale (as defined below) and the Approved Vaccine is purchased for use in an Eligible Country (as defined below), provided that the Designated Supplier commits to supply the Approved Vaccine to Eligible Countries to meet their requirements.[4]
3. Principal Responsibilities of Funder:	Funder will, subject to Sections 7 and 13 below, irrevocably and unconditionally Guarantee that the gross price paid to a Designated Supplier shall be not less than the price set forth in Schedule A (the **"Guaranteed Price"**) for each Qualified Sale of the Approved Vaccine up to the maximum number of sales specified in Schedule A (the **"Approved Maximum"**);[5] provided that (a) the Base Price is not less than the amount specified in Schedule A, and (b) the Approved Vaccine is purchased for use in an Eligible Country. The **"Base Price"** is the amount actually paid, directly or indirectly, by the purchaser of the Approved Vaccine.[6]
4. Principal Responsibilities of Designated Supplier:	The Designated Supplier will (a) use commercially reasonable efforts to create awareness of the availability of the Approved Vaccine in the Eligible Countries in order to meet the public health requirements in the Eligible Countries,[7] (b) [use commercially reasonable efforts to] establish manufacturing capacity for the production of the Approved Vaccine that is sufficient to meet the public health requirements for the Approved Vaccine in the Eligible Countries,[8] (c) obtain and maintain World Health Organization (WHO) prequalification (or any substitute qualification determined by the Committee) for the Approved Vaccine,[9] and those facilities used in its production, as well as any local authorizations and approvals necessary to market and sell the Approved Vaccine in the Eligible Countries, including by complying with all adverse event reporting requirements and providing ongoing evidence of product and production safety and regulatory compliance, (d) provide the Committee with copies of all written communications to or from, including all filings or submissions to, and summaries of all oral communications with, the WHO or any other relevant regulatory agency with respect to the Approved Vaccine, (e) in connection with the marketing, distribution and sale of the Approved Vaccine, comply with the U.S. Foreign Corrupt Practices Act and all other applicable law,[10] (f) provide information as reasonably requested by the Committee from time to time in order to confirm ongoing compliance with the technical specifications and usability requirements set forth in Sections 8 and 9 of the Framework Agreement, (g) agree to be bound by decisions of the Committee acting within the scope of its authority,[11] and (h) continue to supply product to Eligible Countries to meet their requirements as provided in Section 8.

Notes

1. The Framework and Guarantee Agreement term sheets were designed to accommodate a variety of sponsors, despite the fact that there are substantial differences between governmental and nongovernmental organizations in areas such as funding capacity and ability to contractually commit to the Guarantee Agreement. There were discussions regarding mechanisms for ensuring that sponsors are and remain bound by their financial commitments under the Framework and Guarantee Agreements. In the end, the Working Group concluded that traditional commercial mechanisms for ensuring compliance, such as letters of credit or escrow arrangements, would be unattractive to potential Funders as they would result in increased transaction costs and unnecessarily tie up funds that could be made available for more immediate opportunities. Instead, the Working Group elected to implement a bilateral contract structure, which would permit the Developer to pursue standard contract remedies, such as money damages and specific performance, if the Funders fail to satisfy their financial commitments. The Guarantee Agreement term sheet would permit a single Funder, multiple Funders or a system where a lead Funder parcels out participations to sub-Funders. Some of the potential Funders considered by the Working Group include private foundations, developed country governments and international organizations.

2. The Guarantee Agreement is designed so that price for each Qualified Sale could vary. For example, a higher payment could be made in the early years to permit the Developer to recapture R&D costs and capital investments in manufacturing capacity more rapidly, with lower payments in the later years.

3. The Working Group determined that a price Guarantee, rather than a minimum quantity Guarantee, would be the basis for the incentive. See chapter 4 for an explanation. The pricing structure can be designed to provide substantial insurance against demand risk for prospective vaccine developers so as to yield a net present value of revenue comparable with commercial products even under pessimistic uptake scenarios.

4. Sufficient vaccine must be made available to satisfy the requirements of all Eligible Countries. A Developer could not select a few Eligible Countries where it wishes to offer the vaccine or cease to supply vaccine once the price supplements cease to apply.

5. The Approved Maximum and the Guaranteed Price can be set to yield desired revenue. Price guaranties are on a per treatment basis—such as course of immunization—rather than a per dose basis.

6. A Base Price concept, similar to a co-payment, was introduced to create an incentive to help ensure that qualifying vaccines are not wasted and that payments are not made for unusable vaccines. If countries, or other donors, are required to make a minimum investment in an Approved Vaccine, then there is greater likelihood that appropriate quantities of the vaccine will be procured and that those quantities will be administered. This also provides an additional safeguard that donor funds will not be wasted on a vaccine for which there is no market. Especially for diseases for which the vaccine research is still at an early stage, the technical specifications in the Framework Agreement may be established many years in advance of identifying promising vaccine technology, or, for that matter, the delivery of an Approved Vaccine. Intervening events, such as improvements in sanitation or pesticide use, may render a technically adequate vaccine unnecessary. Similarly, unforeseen characteristics of an Approved Vaccine, such as medically harmless but culturally unacceptable side-effects, which would not have been addressed in the technical specifications, may render an otherwise safe vaccine unsuitable in certain countries. The co-payment requirement helps ensure that the advance market

5. Qualified Sale: The sale of the Approved Vaccine for use in an Eligible Country shall be deemed a **"Qualified Sale"** if it meets the criteria set forth in Schedule B, as modified from time to time by the Independent Adjudication Committee. In the event of a conflict between Funder and the Designated Supplier over whether a particular sale of the Approved Vaccine satisfies the criteria for a Qualified Sale, the matter shall be referred to the Independent Adjudication Committee, whose decision shall be final and binding on the parties.

6. Eligible Countries: Each of the countries listed in Schedule C shall be deemed **"Eligible Countries"**). Schedule C may be revised from time to time by the Independent Adjudication Committee in order to (a) add countries whose per capita GDP (as determined by [_____]) is less than [$____], or (b) remove countries whose per capita GDP (as determined by [_____]) is greater than [$____].

7. Cap on Total Commitment [and Termination of Commitment]: The total payment obligation of Funder pursuant to the Guarantee and Supply Agreement, including all payments and distributions to the initial Designated Supplier and any additional or replacement Designated Suppliers, shall (a) not exceed, in the aggregate, [$_____] (the **"Maximum Guaranteed Amount"**), and (b) be subject to termination or modification by the Independent Advisory Committee pursuant to Section 22 of the Framework Agreement. [Schedule C of the Framework Agreement sets forth the assumptions underlying the calculation of the Maximum Guaranteed Amount and the criteria for adjusting it if the number of Eligible Countries is materially reduced or a *force majeure* event occurs.]

8. Supply The Designated Supplier shall supply all requirements of the Approved Vaccines in Eligible Countries during the Funding Term as provided herein and, thereafter, for a period of [10] years, or such longer period as the Designated Supplier may determine (the **"Supply Term"**), at a price not to exceed (a) if the Designated Supplier has received payments for the sale of the Approved Vaccine in Eligible Countries (the **"Gross Sales"**) in amounts, in the aggregate, greater than [$_____] (the **"Minimum Gross Sales Amount"**), then the lesser of [___]% of its fully burdened (without recapture of research and development) costs and expenses to manufacture the Approved Vaccine and [$___] per Dose (as defined in Schedule B), and (b) if the Designated Supplier has not received such payments in such amounts, then the per-Dose amount in clause (a) shall be increased by [___]% only until the aggregate Gross Sales for the Approved Vaccine equals the Minimum Gross Sales Amount, whereupon the increase in this clause (b) shall cease to apply.[12]

commitment will be used for Approved Vaccines that actually meet the requirements of the Eligible Countries.

7. Although the Designated Supplier has responsibility for generating awareness of the availability of Approved Vaccines in Eligible Countries, the Working Group, as noted above, recognized that the Funders must also share in this responsibility.

8. It is critical that the Designated Supplier have adequate manufacturing capacity to meet all of the requirements of the Eligible Countries, not just the Approved Maximum amount of product. The Guarantee Agreement requires that the Designated Supplier use commercially reasonable efforts in this regard, but a higher standard, such as best efforts or an absolute obligation, may be preferable in certain circumstances. In addition, as noted below, consideration needs to be given to the contract remedy if the Designated Supplier fails to establish adequate manufacturing capacity, or otherwise to meet its supply requirements, under the Guarantee Agreement, particularly once the Guaranteed Price commitment has been exhausted.

9. The Working Group recognized that it would be extremely costly to create an Independent Adjudication Committee that was fully capable of evaluating, approving and monitoring the Eligible Vaccines and their ongoing production. Accordingly, the Guarantee Agreement permits the Independent Adjudication Committee to rely on third parties and their procedures, such as the WHO and its prequalification process.

10. Compliance with the Foreign Corrupt Practices Act was imposed to alleviate concern that illegal payments might be used to generate demand. Obviously, the purpose of the advance market commitment is to generate orders for vaccines that will be used, not to simply to generate orders for vaccines.

11. The Working Group recognized the tension between the need for certainty in the determinations of the Independent Adjudication Committee and the need for some review. Court review was deemed impractical in most circumstances. Instead, the goal is to create an IAC that would be viewed as independent by all participants in the Framework, but that is subject to review if it exceeds or abuses its authority, and with respect to certain critical decisions such as a decision to alter or terminate the Funder's payment obligation in the face of a force majeure event, as discussed in note 15 below.

12. The Guarantee Agreement requires that the Designated Supplier continue to make Approved Vaccines available even after the Funding Period expires on a cost-plus basis subject to a cap. If there are multiple Designated Suppliers, the cap will be increased for a limited time for any Designated Supplier that does not receive a certain minimum percentage of the Maximum Guaranteed Amount during the Funding Term, which amount is defined as the Minimum Gross Sales Amount. The increase will cease to be effective, and the cap will return to the predetermined amount, once the Designated Supplier's aggregate sales equal the Minimum Gross Sales Amount. The Minimum Gross Sales Amount is intended to be a rough proxy for a return on the Developer's investment in the Eligible Product, but cannot exceed 100% of the Maximum Guaranteed Amount. For simplicity, the term sheet includes a cost-plus formula, subject to a cap, for determining the ongoing supply price, but it is possible to include more complex hybrid options. For example, a formula could be employed that would allow the Designated Supplier to share in the benefits of reducing the cost of production. In any event, setting the ongoing supply price is a critical component of the advance market commitment.

9. Intellectual Property: The Designated Supplier shall own all right, title and interest in and to the Approved Vaccine; provided, however, if the Designated Supplier fails to supply Approved Vaccine in the Eligible Countries as required in Section 8 during the Funding Term or the Supply Term and, in any event, within 2 years prior to the expiration of the Supply Term, the Designated Supplier shall grant Funder, or its designee, a non-exclusive, irrevocable, perpetual, license (with the right to sublicense) solely to make, have made, use, sell, offer for sale and import the Approved Vaccine in any Eligible Country, but Funder shall not have rights to any other products and shall have no rights outside the Eligible Countries, except the right to make and have made Approved Vaccine for use in Eligible Countries. The license grant shall be royalty-free, unless the Designated Supplier has not been paid the Minimum Gross Sales Amount, in which case such grant shall be subject to a royalty of [___]% of net sales until such time as the aggregate royalty payments to the Designated Supplier equal the product of (a) [___]%, multiplied by (b) the amount, if any, by which the Minimum Gross Sales Amount exceeds the aggregate Gross Sales of the Approved Vaccine, whereupon such vaccine will be fully paid and no further royalties shall be due.[13]

10. Representation and Warranties: [TBD]

11. Indemnification: The Designated Supplier will defend and indemnify the Funder and the members of the Independent Adjudication Committee from all claims and losses arising out of or related to (a) the use of the Approved Vaccine, including claims and losses for physical or mental injury (including death) and (b) infringement or misappropriation of intellectual property.[14]

12. Term: The Guarantee and Supply Agreement shall begin on the date that the Committee designated the first Approved Vaccine and continue through such time as the Maximum Guaranteed Amount has been paid (the **"Funding Term"**), and, thereafter, until the end of the Supply Term, unless earlier terminated pursuant to Section 13.

13. Termination: The Guarantee and Supply Agreement may be terminated by either party in the event of a material breach that is not cured within 30 days of notice thereof from the non-breaching party.

In addition, Funder shall have the right to terminate the Guarantee and Supply Agreement (a) with respect to a particular Designated Supplier in the event the Independent Adjudication Committee determines that the Approved Vaccine of that Designated Supplier no longer satisfies the technical specifications and usability requirements set forth in Sections 8 and 9 of the Framework Agreement, or (b) in the event of a *force majeure* event as determined by the Independent Advisory Committee as set forth in Section 22 of the Framework Agreement.[15]

13. If the Designated Supplier of an Approved Vaccine fails to meet its supply requirements under the Guarantee Agreement, it would be required to grant the Funder, or its designee, a non-exclusive, royalty-free (except as necessary to provide the Designated Supplier with the Minimum Gross Sales Amount, as described above) license to exploit the Approved Vaccine only in Eligible Countries. Although less than ideal, this is intended to make the relevant technology available to the Funder if the Designated Supplier breaches its obligations under the Guarantee Agreement. However, because this provision may not provide much of an incentive not to breach, especially if a Designated Supplier has already received the Maximum Guaranteed Amount and because, even with this license, there could be a disruption of supply, potential Funders may wish to consider other penalties that would disincentivize a Designated Supplier from breaching, such as liquidated damages provisions.

14. Indemnification was deemed to be particularly important to attract qualified members to serve on the Independent Adjudication Committee. It is contemplated that this indemnification would be similar to that which is provided for directors and officers of corporations.

15. A *force majeure* provision permitting the Funder to alter the Guarantee Agreement based upon extraordinary events has been included. The *force majeure* clause would permit the Independent Adjudication Committee to void or alter the Guarantee Agreement in the event of major changes to technology or disease epidemiology that render a vaccine either inappropriate or unnecessary. For example, if advances in pesticides substantially reduced the incidence of malaria in Eligible Countries, then the Funder's financial obligation would be reduced accordingly. As noted in Section 7 of the Guarantee Agreement term sheet, Schedule C would include criteria, such as assumptions underlying the Framework Agreement, to guide the Independent Adjudication Committee in taking any such extraordinary action, which, as noted in the Framework Agreement term sheet, would be subject to review.

14. Addition of New Designated Suppliers:	If the Independent Adjudication Committee determines (by a 2/3 vote of its members and using the standards specified in Schedule B of the Framework Agreement) that a newly developed vaccine is superior to the previously selected Approved Vaccine, whether for certain target populations or epidemiological conditions or otherwise, and the Developer of the newly developed vaccine elects to become a party to the Guarantee Agreement, the Developer of the new vaccine shall be deemed a "Designated Supplier", the new vaccine shall be deemed an "Approved Vaccine" and the new Designated Supplier shall have the right to compete with the original Designated Supplier to make Qualified Sales of the new Approved Vaccine in the Eligible Countries under the Guarantee Agreement.[16] The addition of new Designated Suppliers and Approved Vaccines shall, in each case, be subject to the cap on Sponsor's total commitment set forth in Section 7.
15. Remedies in the Event of Breach:	[TBD]
16. Dispute Resolution:	[Arbitration under AAA rules in NY, NY].
17. Governing Law:	[New York law].
18. Waiver of Immunity:	If the Funder is a sovereign, it will (a) acknowledge that the transactions are subject to private commercial law, and (b) waive sovereign immunity.
19. Other Provisions:	Other covenants, terms and provisions as requested by legal counsel to Funder or the Designated Supplier.

16. The Working Group devoted considerable discussion to the question of whether more than one Developer would be permitted to receive payments under the Guarantee Agreement. On the one hand, the Working Group felt that it was important to preserve incentives for product improvements and that it would be important to use superior products should they be developed. On the other hand, the Working Group was concerned companies might be less willing to risk large investments in early research if they faced the prospect of entry of "me too" products offering no significant advance over the original vaccine. However, many of the industry participants interviewed by the Working Group indicated that they would prefer to have multiple suppliers over a winner-takes-all approach. Recognizing that independent research may lead to the development of substantially similar products, another option would be to permit any qualifying vaccines, whether or not superior, that are tendered within a window (*e.g.,* one year) after the approval of the initial Approved Vaccine to be accepted without showing superiority, provided that the second vaccine resulted from independent research and is not simply a generic copy.

Schedule A to model term sheet for Guarantee and Supply Agreement

Base Price, Guaranteed Price and Approved Maximum

A. Base Price. The minimum Base Price shall be an amount not less than [$__] per Dose (as defined in Schedule B).

B. Guaranteed Price.

C. Approved Maximum (quantity of vaccine in Doses).

Schedule B to model term sheet for Guarantee and Supply Agreement

Criteria for Qualified Sales

A.   Buyer Criteria.

1. Buyers Included. Qualified Buyer include (a) UNICEF, (b) WHO, (c) Pan American Health Organization, (d) any individual Eligible Country that is purchasing for the benefit of the public sector or local nonprofits, and (e) and any other buyer approved by the Independent Adjudication Committee.

2. Buyers Excluded. A pharmaceutical company, acting directly or indirectly thorough one or more intermediaries, shall not qualify as a Qualified Buyer.

B.   Sales Criteria.

1. Course of Treatment. A single course of treatment, regardless of the number of individual immunizations, required to provide the desired efficacy and duration of protection shall be deemed a single "Dose" and shall constitute a single sale. For example, if 3 immunizations over a period of 2 years are required to achieve the desired efficacy and duration of protection, then the sale of all 3 immunizations, one Dose, shall be required to constitute a Qualified Sale.

2. Bundled Sales. In the event that the Designated Supplier bundles the sale of the Approved Vaccine to a purchaser with the sale or licensing of another product or service of the Designated Supplier or its affiliates, the Designated Supplier shall reasonably assign prices to (allocate revenue amounts between) the Approved Vaccine and such other products or services sold or licensed by the Designated Supplier or its affiliates to the purchaser, in accordance with the terms set forth in Exhibit B1 in order to ensure that the Designated Supplier has attributed a reasonable and equitable portion of that sale to the Approved Vaccine.

3. No Top Up. The Designated Supplier shall not seek or receive any additional compensation or value for the sale of the Approved Vaccine in an Eligible Country other than compensation from the purchaser in the form of the Base Price and the compensation from the Funder under the terms of the

Guarantee and Supply Agreement; provided, however, that the Designated Supplier may seek and receive additional compensation or value if (a) additional Funders are added to the Guarantee and Supply Agreement by amendment, or (b) approved by the Independent Adjudication Committee in writing.

4. Use in an Eligible Country. If the Approved Vaccine is purchased for use in a particular Eligible Country, the Designated Supplier must have a reasonable expectation that the Approved Vaccine will actually be used in such Eligible Country. For purposes of illustrating the foregoing, if UNICEF, as it presently operates, certifies that a country has certain requirements for the Approved Vaccine, then the Designated Supplier will have a reasonable expectation that such requirements of the Approved Vaccine will actually be used in such country.

C. Other Criteria.
[*TBD*]

Schedule C to model term sheet for Guarantee and Supply Agreement

Eligible Countries
[*Insert e.g. Vaccine Fund–eligible countries.*]